BETWEEN HIV PREVENTION AND LGBTI RIGHTS

AFRICAN PERSPECTIVES

Kelly Askew, Laura Fair, and Pamila Gupta
Series Editors

Between HIV Prevention and LGBTI Rights

The Political Economy of Queer Activism in Ghana

Ellie Gore

University of Michigan Press
Ann Arbor

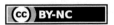
For questions or permissions, please contact um.press.perms@umich.edu

Published in the United States of America by the
University of Michigan Press
Manufactured in the United States of America
Printed on acid-free paper
First published October 2024

A CIP catalog record for this book is available from the British Library.

Library of Congress Control Number: 2024016790

ISBN 978-0-472-07702-1 (hardcover : alk. paper)
ISBN 978-0-472-05702-3 (paper : alk. paper)
ISBN 978-0-472-90478-5 (open access ebook)

DOI: https://doi.org/10.3998/mpub.12067615

This work was supported by the UK's Economic and Social Research Council (grant number ES/S011722/1).

The University of Michigan Press's open access publishing program is made possible thanks to additional funding from the University of Michigan Office of the Provost and the generous support of contributing libraries.

Since I conducted the fieldwork for this research in 2013, a number of the activists I met, some of whom participated in this study, have sadly and tragically passed away. I feel privileged to have met them and witnessed their bravery, humor, and solidarity. This book is dedicated to them.

CONTENTS

ACKNOWLEDGMENTS

This book would not have been possible without the support of the many peer educators and activists I met in Ghana. I am particularly indebted to Samuel Azumah Nelson, who assisted me with many aspects of the fieldwork and data collection, and to the executive directors and staff of the two NGOs that allowed me to volunteer with them and to observe the work of their organizations. I owe sincere thanks to Serena Dankwa and Akua Gyamerah for their scholarship and for the conversations we have had about queer politics in Ghana over the years. I am also incredibly grateful for the feedback and encouragement I received from colleagues at the University of Sheffield while I was working on this manuscript, especially Genevieve LeBaron, Natalie Langford, Tom Hunt, Merisa Thompson, and Liam Stanley, who all read chapter drafts and generously shared their time and expertise. I was also inspired by the intellectual community of postdocs at the University of Sheffield, especially Merve Sancak, Nabeela Ahmed, and Caroline Metz.

I am indebted to my doctoral supervisors at the University of Birmingham, Emma Foster and Martin Rew, for their sage advice throughout every stage of the PhD process. I would also like to thank Nicola Smith, who first pointed me in the direction of feminist political economy and who has since provided much intellectual inspiration, as well as words of encouragement. Since the timeline of this project has been long (!), I have also benefited from the support of new colleagues at the University of Manchester, particularly Adrienne Roberts, who spurred me on when I was threatening to abandon the project at the final hurdle. I owe further thanks to the editors and editorial board at the University of Michigan Press, as well as the anonymous readers, whose thoughtful feedback and suggestions have resulted in a vastly improved manuscript. I am also grateful to the photographer Eric Gyamfi for giving me permission to use one of his images for the front cover of this book. Finally, I would like to thank George Aidoo and Joseph Mills from African Bureau Limited, whose knowledge and expertise in the languages and culture of Ghana were invaluable.

This research was generously supported by the UK's Economic and Social Research Council through a PhD scholarship and postdoctoral fellowship (ES/S011722/1), and through their open access longform publication fund.

Some of the ideas and arguments advanced in the book were developed through writing published previously as journal articles. The prologue draws on "Reflexivity and Queer Embodiment: Some Reflections on Sexualities Research in Ghana," *Feminist Review* 120, no. 1 (2018), 101–119; Chapter 1 draws on "Understanding Queer Oppression and Resistance in the Global Economy: Towards a Theoretical Framework for Political Economy," *New Political Economy* 27, no. 2 (2022), 296–311; and Chapter 3 draws on "The political economy of HIV prevention in Ghana: peer education, queer social reproductive labor, and the global development industry," *International Feminist Journal of Politics*, 26, no. 2, 306–28 (2024). I am grateful for the publishers' permission to publish revised material based on this work.

I definitely would not have finished this project without the love and encouragement of my friends and family, who have been there through the many ups and downs of life over the past decade: Lydia Stober, Aeryn Priyanu, Leona Chaliha, Jessie Maryon Davies, Esme Wilson, Milly Oldfield, Jo Tyabji, and Lou Mulcahy provided lots of laughter, as well as emotional (and occasionally material) support throughout my PhD and beyond; Chardine Taylor-Stone, whose political insights and general cheerleading sustained me through the writing process; my parents, Van and Jill Gore, who have supported me in so many ways and who have enthusiastically read everything I have ever written since the age of five (well, mainly my dad); and my sister, Jo Gore, who I am lucky to call my best friend as well as my sister.

PROLOGUE

Freedom is not something that one people can bestow on another as a gift. They claim it as their own and none can keep it from them.
  —Kwame Nkrumah, July 10, 1953, speech in the House of Commons, London

Always ally yourself with those on the bottom, on the margins, and at the periphery of the centers of power. And in so doing, you will land yourself at the very center of some of the most important struggles of our society and our history.
  —Barbara Ransby, "Fortieth Anniversary of the Combahee River Collective Statement" (2017:183)

I first observed the growing politicization of homosexuality in Ghana in 2011, when I was working for an NGO in the Upper East Region of the country. In May of that year, newspaper reports that "8,000 homosexuals" had "registered" with HIV charities in the Western and Central Regions provoked outcry within media and political spheres (Daily Graphic 2011). The MP for the Western Region, Paul Evans Aidoo, called for homosexuals to be "rounded up" and expelled, labelling homosexuality "abominable" and a "canker" that had no place in Ghanaian society (MyJoyOnline 2011). I recall my work colleagues, who had seldom mentioned homosexuality prior to this time, discussing the reports with great interest. Although not everyone agreed, much of the discussion focused on a perceived clash between Ghanaian cultural values and the teachings of the Bible on the one hand, and homosexual practices on the other. These arguments mirrored contemporary media reporting and commentary, which frequently depicted homosexuality as "un-Ghanaian" and "un-Christian," a threat to public health and morality.[1]

The UK prime minister, David Cameron, stirred up controversy again later in the same year when he threatened to withdraw aid funding from African countries with a "poor track record" on gay rights, such as Ghana and Uganda (BBC 2011). Cameron told reporters he had raised the issue with the Commonwealth Heads of Government and emphasized that countries in receipt of development aid must adhere to "proper human rights." Cameron's interventions elicited a defiant response from Ghana's then president, John

Atta Mills, who declared that the United Kingdom had "no right to tell Ghana what to do" (Gray 2011). The United Kingdom's interventions were also criticized by a number of prominent Ghanaian religious leaders, with the general overseer of the Evangelical Church speaking out to denounce gay rights as "wicked" (Jalulah and Freiku 2011).

Like the HIV news story, Cameron's comments sparked fierce debate among many of my Ghanaian colleagues and friends: a mix of religious and moral objections to homosexuality, anti-imperial sentiment, and assertions of political, cultural, and economic sovereignty. These responses capture some of the complex issues that imbue debates over the so-called gay question (Osei 2018) in the contemporary Ghanaian state. Yet I felt like one key part of this picture was missing: Where were the voices of Ghana's queer communities and activist organizations? What did they make of the British government's stance? Skimming through internet articles on the Cameron controversy, I came across a letter written by a collective of African social justice activists that offered some answers to my questions. The letter criticized the British prime minister for disregarding the concerns and strategies of activists working on these issues on the ground and for stoking up hostility and resentment toward LGBTI individuals across the continent. One of the signatories of the letter was the Centre for Popular Education and Human Rights Ghana (CEPEHRG), a community NGO working on HIV and sexual rights for "marginalized populations" in Accra. On its website, I found implicit references to CEPEHRG's involvement in LGBTI rights work, accompanied by the simple statement, "Sexual rights are a human right."

Eighteen months later, I traveled to Accra to meet with staff members from CEPEHRG for a research project on activism and politicized homophobia. It took me some time to find their offices, which were located in a sleepy suburb of Accra, quite a distance from the city center. "There is no such thing as a gay rights movement in Ghana," CEPEHRG's assistant director, Charles Yeboah, told me emphatically, before we had even started our interview.[2] I pondered the motivations behind Charles's statement. Perhaps he was growing tired of answering questions from white Western researchers with a newfound interest in gay rights in Africa. Or perhaps he was asserting a difference between Ghanaian activism and the kind of LGBTI activism found in countries like the United Kingdom. Whatever the reason, I felt like he was cautioning me not to exaggerate the scale or scope of activism in the country.

During our interview, I asked Charles about the factors shaping the politicization of homosexuality within the Ghanaian public sphere. Like many of the activists I met subsequently, he identified 2006 as a key turning point in the process of politicization, when reports that a two-day "international gay conference" would take place in Accra appeared in Ghanaian news media. Charles showed me newspaper cuttings from the time, taken from Ghana's leading national newspaper, the *Daily Graphic*. They included reports and editorials criticising the conference and espousing vehement and occasionally violent anti-gay sentiment. It was, he noted, a scary time to be involved in LGBTI rights work and CEPEHRG was caught off guard by the level of attention the story attracted. Leading political and religious leaders responded angrily to the reports and the minister for information and national orientation, Kwamena Bartels, publicly condemned the conference on the grounds that it offended "the culture, morality and heritage of the entire people of Ghana" (BBC 2006). While the exact origins of the conference rumor are hard to ascertain, activists pinpoint remarks made in a radio debate by Prince Macdonald, a spokesperson for the Gay and Lesbian Association of Ghana (GALAG), as the source of the story and trigger of the backlash. According to CEPEHRG staff, the "homoconference" rumor was a deliberate misrepresentation of a planned HIV conference, which was used by the media to target activists and stir up homophobia.[3] In the aftermath of the controversy, GALAG released a statement clarifying the circumstances surrounding the conference rumor:

> The Gay and Lesbian Association of Ghana feels compelled to issue this statement in the face of mounting misinformation being made public in both print and electronic media about an alleged two-day international gay conference, supposedly coming on in Accra International Conference Centre and in Koforidua, respectively. We wish to clarify . . . as an association, we are not prepared to organize such a conference anywhere in Ghana, let alone any part of the universe, at this point.[4]

RESEARCHING QUEER ACTIVISM

Charles's statement, "There is no such thing as a gay rights movement in Ghana," rung in my ears as I prepared for a much longer period of research exploring HIV initiatives and LGBTI rights activism in Ghana in 2013, on which this book is based. He had, in a sense, anticipated some of the central questions of my inquiry: What is the character of queer political activism in Ghana? How do activists conceptualize LGBTI rights and queer struggle? And if a social movement optic is not appropriate for understanding queer activism, what is?

One of the challenges of researching activism in the Ghanaian context is the relatively limited number of (formal) actors involved and, relatedly, the often discreet and non-confrontational approaches adopted by queer individuals and groups seeking to challenge injustice. This has been conceptualized by the lawyers and activists Anthony Olouch and Monica Tabengwa (2017) as the "double-edged sword" of visibility, which refers to the challenges and dilemmas facing activists in climates marked by pervasive forms of political, cultural, and religious homophobia. Put otherwise, strategic decisions over the degree and character of visibility adopted by activists are critical in contexts where it is dangerous to be out, but where being out is simultaneously construed as an important way of "demystifying" queer subjectivities and pushing demands for LGBTI rights up the political agenda (Olouch and Tabengwa 2017; see also Currier 2012).

Questions of visibility are also of practical concern to scholars engaged in the study of queer politics and activism in Africa. The still emergent corpus of primary research on queer activism in West Africa therefore reflects, in part, the repressive political and legal contexts that govern homosexuality in some parts of the region, including Ghana, which act as a constraint on or deterrent to academic inquiry.[5] During my research in 2013, for example, I encountered a number of individuals who had begun and subsequently abandoned studies of queer politics in Ghana (and other parts of Africa) due to concerns over safety. Things have changed in many ways in the intervening decade, not least with the growing establishment of "queer African studies" as an interdisciplinary field of inquiry (Nyeck 2020). In terms of the academic literature, there is now a rich and wide-ranging body of research on queer African sexualities, subjectivities, and politics (see, for example, collections by Ekine and Abbas 2013; Nyeck and Epprecht 2013; Matebeni 2014; Sandfort et al. 2015; Matebeni et al. 2018; Nyeck 2020), as well as growing representation of queer African perspectives in the field of culture and the arts.[6] The tendency for studies of queer politics to focus on southern Africa (see, for example, Epprecht 2004; Morgan and Wieringa 2005; Currier 2012; Swarr 2012; Matebeni 2014; Lorway 2014) has also been increasingly redressed. In the Ghanaian context, Anima Adjepong's (2021) ethnography of "Afropolitanism" explores the transnational politics of identity and belonging among middle-class Ghanaians, with a particular focus on (queer) sexuality. Elsewhere, social anthropological work by Serena Dankwa (2021) and Kwame Edwin Otu (2022) has addressed the lacuna of scholarship on the everyday intimacies of queer working-class sexualities in Ghana, which, as Dankwa notes, "exist alongside and beyond sexual rights politics" (2021:19). Although these studies differ in their disciplinary orientations and contributions, the authors are careful to explore how their own queer subject positions, both in the diaspora and "at home", relate to their respective topics of inquiry.

Against this background, it would be difficult and, I think, ill-advised to write a book about queer activism in Ghana without accounting for positionality, especially as a white, queer British researcher. Feminist scholars have long prioritized practices of reflexivity in academic inquiry, as part of a broader attempt to interrogate the politics of power, voice, and subjectivity (Harding 1987; Spivak 1988; Minh-Ha 1989; Haraway 1991; Behar 1996). Gayatri Spivak (1988) made a landmark intervention into these debates with her essay "Can the Subaltern Speak?" In this paper, Spivak examines the constitution of the subaltern subject within Western academic writing, using a conversation between Gilles Deleuze and Michel Foucault as a starting point. Spivak questions the universalist ideas and ideological biases that underpin the authors' invocation of the "workers' struggle" and shows why this invocation is inadequate to capture the differentiated global character of the capitalist economy, particularly unequal center-periphery relations. Thus, she suggests, even those "intellectuals who are the best prophets of heterogeneity and the Other" continue to reinscribe the West as Subject (Spivak 1988:67).

Writing within the African feminist tradition, Oyèrónké Oyěwùmí (1997) offers a similarly coruscating critique of the state of Western academic scholarship, in this instance surveying the impact of Western theories on "African subjects." She argues that "academics have become one of the most effective international hegemonizing forces, producing not homogenous social experiences but a homogeny of hegemonic forces" (Oyěwùmí 1997:16). For Oyěwùmí, Western theorizing, including Western feminism, operates from a set of universalizing and ethnocentric assumptions, particularly regarding gender and the body, which work to reify and reinforce power asymmetries. Sylvia Tamale (2020:4) summarizes these dynamics succinctly as "Western coloniality, hegemony and dominance in knowledge production." What this means, inter alia, is that the problem is not only presently one of epistemology—about how knowledge is produced in the contemporary juncture—but is deeply embedded within the history of academic inquiry itself. As the Indigenous scholar Linda Tuhiwai Smith (1999:1) points out,

"The "term 'research' is inextricably linked to European imperialism and colonialism."

These wide-ranging critiques, as advanced by Black, Indigenous, and other feminist scholars of color, problematize the act of speaking for, with, or about the "Other," the theoretical and conceptual tools that academics in the Global North use to narrativize their subjects, and the past and present power relations these practices uphold. Such acts of representation are particularly loaded for (white) Euro-American scholars of African sexualities, given how colonial constructions—which include characterizing Africa (and African sexualities) as "primitive," "pathological" and "libidinously eroticized"— have continued to shape hegemonic ways of knowing about the continent (McClintock 1995: 22; Arnfred 2004; Tamale 2011).[7] This is why Jane Soothill, in discussing "the burden of history" and her own positionality as a white Western woman writing about Ghana, acknowledges that Africa represents the "'Other' *par excellence* of the Western world" (2007:21).[8]

I do not take these critiques lightly. Indeed, I have spent a number of years wondering whether I should write this book at all. There is no doubt that, in a context like Ghana, it is impossible to separate my whiteness (and my "Britishness") from my activities as a researcher (and from my embodiment as a queer person). My positionality is thus constituted by the "burden of history," to use Soothill's phrase, but also by contemporary socioeconomic inequalities and geopolitical power relations. As Jemima Pierre (2012) explains in her book *The Predicament of Blackness*, Ghana's sizeable population of expatriate workers, their association with wealth and technological superiority, and their location within Ghana's wider political economy structures a "discourse of whiteness" that reflects and reinforces global white supremacy. These local/global processes are rooted in historic and contemporary structures of racial domination, which trace from Ghana's colonial past through to the neoliberal present. While Pierre (2012) notes that these formations are shifting and contested, for example, through the Ghanaian government's reformulation of pan-Africanist ideology and "celebration of Blackness," she underlines the continuing power of white racial privilege in the postcolonial Ghanaian state.

I should acknowledge too that my queerness worked, in some ways, to bring me closer to the people I was studying, insofar as we could identify shared experiences of homophobia and, perhaps, shared recognition of what it means to transgress hegemonic sexual and gender norms. Yet this experiential commonality was at best fleeting, since the disciplinary power of heteronormativity may transcend axes of difference such as race and class, but these very same axes continue to constitute its character and effects. In other words, my experiences as a queer person are a far cry from the stories of violence and oppression recounted by the queer working-class men who participated in my research: accounts of physical and sexual violence, familial rejection, homelessness, poor health, poverty, and stigmatization. My attempt to recognize commonality and difference is therefore not intended to downplay the significance of racial hierarchies and class relations, material inequalities and colonial legacies, or the power of the researcher in representing other people's voices. Rather, it speaks to the ontological impossibility of separating out axes of gender, race, class, sexuality, and nationality; I will always be embodied as a white person in Ghana, with all the historic and contemporary power and privilege that entails. *And* I move through the world as a queer person and, with that, bring some understanding of what it means to live outside society's "regimes of the normal" (Warner 1993:xxvi).

Throughout this book, I seek to acknowledge these dynamics and tensions and to position myself explicitly in the field of research, without, I hope, decentering the lives and experiences of the queer men who comprise the heart of this study. I imagine that some readers will remain unconvinced by these efforts or will question the fundamental integrity of such a project given the ongoing material and epistemological inequities that shape the academic study of "Africa." I acknowledge these critiques, but, as a queer, socialist, and feminist scholar, I am ultimately inclined to believe that we must move beyond recognizing our own positionality to consider how these insights might be engaged in practical ways and, in the words of Chandra Mohanty, to "practice solidarity across difference" (2003). For Mohanty (2003:223), this means that "cross-cultural feminist work must be attentive to the micropolitics of context, subjectivity, and struggle, as well as the macropolitics of global economic and political systems and processes." Attentiveness to both the micro- and macropolitical, to linking the personal to the political economic, is a core aim of this book. In this, I am also inspired by the transgender scholar and activist Leslie Feinberg (1992:6), who argued that "solidarity is built on understanding how and why oppression exists and who profits from it." It is with the practice of solidarity in mind that I present this book.

Introduction

They kept on saying we are not here. But of late, we are here.
—David Kato, *They Will Say We Are Not Here* (2012)

Sexual health and sexual rights have become increasingly mainstream concerns within global development discourse over the past three decades. The global HIV epidemic has been a key driver in this shift, compelling donor governments, development agencies, international organizations, and civil society actors to address matters of sexuality and to invest extensively in sexual and reproductive health programs across the Global South. With queer men—or "men who have sex with men" (MSM) in epidemiological parlance—bearing a disproportionate burden of the disease in Africa, rights-based health interventions have sought to tackle the epidemic by bringing together, educating, and "empowering" queer African communities. This book explores the impacts of these interventions on the lives and political activities of queer activists in the West African country of Ghana.

Scholars have typically differentiated between "human rights" and "public health" approaches to LGBTI rights in development discourse, sometimes also referred to as a divide between "public health" and "rights activism" (Epprecht 2013) or "social justice" and "public health" approaches (Currier and McKay 2017). In contrast, this book uses the term "sexual health rights" to capture the extent to which these approaches have converged and coalesced at the level of development policy and practice in Ghana.[1] This coming together is evident in national and key stakeholder policy documents pertaining to HIV prevention, as well as the political and programmatic orientation of Ghana's longest-running LGBTI/HIV organizations. For the purposes of this book, I focus on sexual health rights initiatives tied to HIV prevention for MSM, which, in the Ghanaian context, primarily entail improving access to healthcare services, such as HIV testing and counselling, enhancing knowledge of HIV and STIs, promoting behavioral changes, such as condom usage, and other community empowerment interventions. These sexual health rights initiatives provide the cornerstone of development's overarching sexual rights agenda.

Within donor circles, Ghana is often hailed as one of West Africa's success stories. Dubbed a "star pupil" by the World Bank for its approach to structural adjustment (Hutchful 1995), the country has recorded relatively consistent patterns of economic growth and substantial decreases in poverty levels over the past three decades (Aryeetey and Fenny 2017). However, improvements in macroeconomic indicators and national poverty levels belie a number of more problematic trends: significant spatial and gender disparities in income and employment levels; widespread informalization; uneven access to health, education, and other basic services; high rates of youth unemployment; and growing economic inequalities. These inequalities are especially pronounced between Ghana's northern and southern regions and within large cities, such as Accra and Kumasi (Obeng-Odoom 2012). At the time of writing in 2023, a perfect storm of currency depreciation, surging inflation, energy crisis, and high levels of government indebtedness further threatens Ghana's fragile shoots of economic growth.[2]

Perhaps nowhere are these structural contradictions and economic divides more apparent than the capital city, Accra. Taking a tour of the central commercial district of Osu, it is hard to miss the hallmarks of neoliberal economic globalization. The streets are lined with telecommunication stores such as Vodafone and Tigo, there is a KFC restaurant and several South African–owned fast food chains, and a towering shopping mall sells imported goods at inflated prices. A steady stream of SUVs chokes the central traffic artery of Oxford Street. Mercedes, Range Rovers, Toyota V8s—the status symbols du jour of Accra's expanding middle-class and expat populations—jostle for space alongside the city's battered *trotros* and white and yellow taxis.[3] Further afield, in the city's wealthy suburbs of East Legon, Labone, Cantonments, and Airport Residential, are the homes of the Ghanaian elites, where businessmen, politicians, NGO workers, foreign developers, and other beneficiaries of the private enterprise boom live in gated complexes, guarded by security and barbed wire.

Step off Osu's main drag of Oxford Street, however, and the cramped, crumbling compound houses, overflowing drains, piles of uncollected rubbish, and throngs of hawkers, street food vendors, and *kayayei* tell a very different story of neoliberal economic development in Ghana.[4] *Kayayei*, predominantly young women and girls who have migrated from the country's northern regions in search of jobs, walk the streets for hours on end, selling bananas, groundnuts, pineapple, pawpaw, or avocados. Under the relentless equatorial sun, this is exhausting work that is likely to earn just a few Ghana cedis per day.

This book is about queer activism. But I begin with this vignette of Accra for a number of reasons. Having spent over a decade of my life working in Ghana, it strikes me that these sharp contrasts can become blunted amid the routine and the familiarity of the everyday. Yet, as this book goes on to argue, it is this socioeconomic landscape, these particular material conditions, that so profoundly mediate queer working-class lives. It is here too, among the traders and the *trotro* passengers, the hawkers and the hustlers, that Accra's working-class queers can be found, caught up, like many others, in the daily struggle for survival. These dynamics have far-reaching ramifications for how working-class queers experience oppression, for their understandings of rights and resistance, and for the broader character and contours of queer Ghanaian activism, as it is (re)shaped by global development initiatives on HIV. Understanding these dynamics, I argue, requires us to grapple with fundamental problems of political economy; structure and agency; production and social reproduction; class exploitation and hierarchies of race, gender, sexuality, and citizenship; and patterns of uneven development, which are not only rooted in contemporary dynamics in the global economy, but in the "afterlives" of slavery and colonialism.[5]

THE POLITICIZATION OF HOMOSEXUALITY IN GHANA

Homosexuality has become increasingly politicized in Ghana over the past twenty years.[6] In 2006, newspaper reports that an "international gay conference" was being organized in Accra prompted outcry among leading political and religious figures (BBC 2006). This controversy marked the first in a series of public flashpoints—what I term in this book moral panics—over homosexuality in the West African state. This climate of panic and politicized homophobia continues today: in February 2021, a newly opened LGBTI community center in Accra was shut down by the Ghanaian police, following outcry from journalists, politicians, and religious leaders (Akinwotu 2021). A few months later in May 2021, the Ghanaian police arrested twenty-one people attending a workshop on human rights violations against LGBTI people in Ho, the capital of the Volta region.[7]

Under Ghana's "unnatural carnal knowledge" law, the origins of which date back to the era of British colonialism, sexual relations between men are criminalized. "Unnatural carnal knowledge" is classified as a misdemeanor and carries a prison sentence of up to three years. In June 2021, an "anti-LGBTQ+" bill, formally called the Promotion of Proper Human Sexual Rights and Ghanaian Family Values Bill, was proposed within the Ghanaian parliament. This bill would significantly strengthen and expand the law's existing anti-LGBTI provisions, notably by proscribing "LGBTQ+ and related activities," including "propaganda," "advocacy for," and "promotion" thereof, on the grounds that "they do not accord with the sociocultural values of any ethnic group in Ghana."[8] The proposal of the bill reflects an intensification of anti-LGBTI politics at the state level in Ghana and forms part of a broader trajectory whereby homosexuality has become politicized within the West African state, which has transmuted into increasingly strident forms of "politicized homophobia" (Currier 2018).[9]

This process of politicization has been driven by a multifaceted set of factors at the domestic and global level, which include prominent Ghanaian religious and political leaders and organizations who mobilize homophobic propaganda and rhetoric, along with key parts of the mainstream media (Mohammed 2020; Asante 2020); multiscalar HIV response that has increased the visibility of MSM as a biomedical population in Ghana; burgeoning domestic human rights activism from NGOs and other community groups working on HIV, MSM, and/or LGBTI issues; growing interest in the global politics of LGBTI rights among key development actors, global governance institutions, and Western governments; and a wider context in which the rise of populist radical-right politics has shaped and accompanied the mobilization of a transnational "anti-gender" movement. This movement comprises a heterogeneous alliance of actors and forces that oppose so-called gender ideology and aim to roll back "progressive legislation won in the last decades by both LGBTQI and feminist movements" (Butler 2021). Within this alliance, the US Christian Right has attracted attention for its role in promoting anti-LGBTI politics and an agenda of expanded criminalization in Africa. By establishing political and economic links, as well as religious ones, with prominent African clerics and churches, conservative US evangelicals warn of the moral dangers of homosexuality. This forms part of what Kapya Kaoma (2009) calls a "globalization of the culture wars," in which new geopolitical dividing lines are being drawn based on matters of sexuality and LGBTI rights.[10]

As this brief overview suggests, the emergence of pervasive forms of politicized homophobia in Ghana has been shaped not only by relations at the state and suprastate levels, but also by the activities of activists, NGOs, and other grassroots organizations. In order to explore these dynamics, this book focuses on what I term the first wave of activist groups that emerged in the late 1990s, during which time a small number of NGOs began working on LGBTI rights and/or HIV prevention among MSM, both in the capital Accra and in other cities such as Takoradi. The growth of sexual rights-based initiatives in Ghana are related to increases in global development funding to tackle the HIV epidemic, as well as significant shifts in Ghanaian public health policy. In this context—and ostensibly in contrast to its politicized stance on homosexuality—the Ghanaian government has worked with local, national, and global development actors to develop targeted interventions for those most at risk of HIV, notably MSM and female sex workers (Gyamerah 2021). At a microlevel, rights-based sexual health interventions have typically been operationalized through peer education programs, in which queer men are recruited by local NGOs to carry out HIV prevention work among their peers.

ABOUT THIS BOOK

This book argues that global development initiatives to promote sexual rights are failing to benefit queer men in Ghana. Against a backdrop of legal repression, politicized homophobia, and everyday violence, poor and working-class queer men struggle to find stable work and housing, face rejection from family and friends, and are more likely to engage in sex work and other transactional sexual relations. This, in turn, puts them at greater risk of HIV, alcohol and substance abuse, ill health, and, ultimately, premature death. These are not isolated trends but are echoed in the lived experience of queer men across parts of the African continent where homosexuality remains criminalized and/or highly stigmatized (Korhonen et al. 2018; Scheibe et al. 2014; Fay et al. 2011; Abara and Garba 2015; Johnson et al. 2010; Baral et al. 2009).[11] To support this argument, the book advances four interrelated lines of analysis. First, it shows that development's overwhelming focus on HIV has shifted the goalposts for queer activists in Ghana, engendering the formalization and NGO-ization of activism and drawing some of the key activist groups that emerged in the late 1990s away from more grassroots forms of organizing.

Second, it explores how global development policies and practices relating to sexual rights work in top-down, technocratic, and managerialist ways that disconnect formal LGBTI/HIV organizations from the communities they are supposed to represent. Third, it locates NGO-led HIV prevention and sexual rights programs within a neoliberal empowerment paradigm in development. In practice, the book argues, this paradigm relies on and exploits the unpaid labor of queer working-class men, reinforces class divides, and individualizes and depoliticizes queer struggle. Fourth and finally, the book shows that development agendas based on sexual health rights simply do not reflect the concerns and priorities of working-class queer communities, which are as much about tackling poverty, unemployment, and economic injustice as they are about addressing specifically sexual rights. In this way, development is not only neglecting the structural roots and facets of queer oppression in Ghana—the nexus of heteronormativity, state-sanctioned repression and violence, and economic exploitation—it is reinforcing and (re)producing them.

Before I go on, a few caveats. The arguments set out in this book are not coming from a place of "Afro-pessimism."[12] Nor should they be used to bolster stereotypical notions of "one homophobic Africa" (Awondo et al. 2012) or to reproduce what Sibongile Ndashe (2013) calls "the single story of 'African homophobia.'" Transnational media discourses on African homophobia frequently traffic in narratives of "queer African 'victimage'" (Currier and Migraine-George 2016:281), which deny agency to queer activists and communities and obscure the heterogenous realities of queer lived experience.[13] Rather, the book aims to be attentive to the specificities of the Ghanaian context, to avoid reduction and generalization, and, above all, to centralize the voices and experiences of queer Ghanaians involved in HIV prevention, LGBTI rights advocacy, and other forms of queer community organizing. I am similarly cognizant of African feminists' long-standing call for scholars to study sexual pleasure, eroticism, and desire, as opposed to reiterating "tired polemics of violence, disease, and reproduction" in the African context (Tamale 2011:31; see also McFadden 2003; Reddy et al. 2018). This injunction evidently informs the fine-grained ethnographic work on queer sexualities in Ghana produced by Dankwa (2021) and Otu (2022). However, given the book's focus on the power relations that constitute global development initiatives on HIV and broader patterns of global economic transformation, and, indeed, with a number of the men I met in 2013 having since passed away, the book necessarily tells a story of structural violence as well as resistance, of oppression as well as struggle.[14] Like Rahul Rao (2020), I understand these dynamics to be fundamentally transnational in character and, moreover, to be rooted in the *longue durée* of colonial and capitalist political economy. Theoretically, I use a queer political economy approach to parse some of the entanglements between (neo)colonialism, imperialism, and neoliberal development processes in the postcolonial juncture and to consider how these contestations come to be played out, and inscribed upon, queer subjectivities and bodies.

A QUEER POLITICAL ECONOMY APPROACH

A number of studies of queer activism in Africa have drawn on political economy (see, for example, Thomann 2014; Thoreson 2014; Hildebrandt and Chua 2017; Currier and McKay 2017; Rao 2020) and there is an established body of scholarship on the political economy of HIV in the African context (see, for example, O'Manique 2004; Nattrass 2014; Nguyen 2010; Hickel 2012; Harman 2015; O'Laughlin 2015; Kenworthy 2017). As far as I am aware, however, no studies to date have advanced a specifically political economy approach to the study of queer oppression and resistance in Africa. In order to explain the value of this approach, the book draws on feminist and queer political economy scholarship, which aims to move beyond what Isabella Bakker and Stephen Gill term "a narrow ontology of states and markets" (2003:4) to centralize how gender and sexuality constitute the global capitalist economy (Gibson-Graham 1996; Hennessy 2000; Peterson 2003; Jacobs and Klesse 2013; Smith 2020). Feminists and other critical scholars have long challenged the state-centric and productivist biases of orthodox political economy (Waylen 1997, 2006; Peterson 2003; Bakker 2007; Steans and Tepe-Belfrage 2008) and highlighted how states and markets are gendered and racialized structures (Elson 1999; Peterson 2003, 2021; Bhattacharya 2017; Bhattacharyya 2018; Tilley and Shilliam 2018). This scholarship has rendered visible the vital contributions made by households and social reproductive labor, which is disproportionately carried out by women (and particularly women of color), to the global economy (Davis 1981; Mies 1986; Glenn 1992; Federici 2004; Bakker 2007; Hoskyns and Rai 2007; LeBaron 2010). In the study of globalization, scholars have further documented the wide-ranging and transformative impacts of economic and social development processes on gender norms, governance practices, and modalities of women's work and activism across the Global South (Elson 1993; Rai 2002; Parpart et al. 2002; Benería 2003; Rai and Waylen 2008; Bair 2010; Mezzadri, Newman, and Stevano 2022).

When it comes to struggles over sexuality, feminist scholars of political economy have typically focused on issues such as sexual violence (Federici 2004; True 2012; Meger 2016; Elias and Rai 2019), sex work (Fortunati 1995; Agathangelou 2006; Kotiswaran 2011; Berg 2021), and/or forms of sexualized inequality relating to biological reproduction, child care, and the care economy (Parreñas 2000; Ehrenreich and Hochschild 2002; Arat-Koç 2006; Fraser 2016). While this literature has increasingly expanded its analysis of sexual struggles beyond the Global North, it tends to understand (cis and heterosexual) women to be the primary subject of analysis when it comes to body politics and therefore (cis and heterosexual) women's sexuality to be the primary object of investigation.[15] This book opens up new directions in this scholarship by examining the impact of development interventions relating to HIV and sexual rights on queer politics and activism in Ghana and on the lives and political activities of queer working-class men. In so doing, it responds to calls to better integrate a queer sensibility into analyses of global capitalism, that is, to "queer" political economy (Smith 2018; see also Cornwall 1997), as well as efforts to "queer" development (Jolly 2000; Lind 2010; Kapoor 2015).[16] One key aspect of this queering entails examining the relationship between queer subjectivities, body politics, and everyday forms of resistance, on the one hand, and macrolevel political economic relations, modes of governance, and trajectories of capitalist crisis, on the other. As Nicola Smith puts it, it means investigating "how the structural inequalities of global capitalism are reproduced in and through intimate, embodied social relations" (2018:106). Another key aspect of this, I argue, entails understanding how contestations over queer sexuality play out in contexts beyond the Global North, against a backdrop of neoliberal economic restructuring and ongoing forms of imperial violence and dispossession.

In order to approach this project, the book brings together insights from feminist political economy with a wider interdisciplinary set of literatures that I term the "social movement," "globalization," and "queering development" frames, as well as radical, queer, and feminist scholarship from Africa and across the diaspora. Based on this, I advance a political economy analysis of queer oppression and resistance in Ghana that illuminates the complex encounters between politicized homophobia, HIV and sexual health rights initiatives, social and economic development processes, and formal and informal strands of queer activism in the contemporary Ghanaian state. Put simply, this approach examines the material consequences of global development processes—as these are constituted by broader dynamics within the global capitalist economy—for queer lives and politics in Ghana. At the same time, it aims to show why the types of oppression and exploitation experienced by minoritized sexual and gendered individuals are not incidental or external to the global capitalist economy, but are (re)productive of it. For the purposes of this book, I operationalize my political economy approach by looking across three thematic areas or dimensions: (1) capitalism, sexuality, and the state; (2) capitalism, sexuality, and global governance (in this context global development policies and practices relating to HIV and sexual rights); and (3) the everyday political economies of queer lives and resistance. I explain this approach in detail in Chapter 2.

Theoretically, the book argues that studies of queer activism in Africa should prioritize questions of political economy. This means paying close attention to the structural contexts in which homophobia and oppression are rooted and enacted and the political economic power relations that constitute queer lives and resistance. It also involves focusing on the materiality of queer oppression and injustice, as this is bound up in the unequal distribution of power, wealth, and resources within the global economy. To do this, I center my analysis on the global development industry, namely aid funding flows and mechanisms, dominant development agendas, norms, and practices, and the infrastructures of HIV response, and link this to broader processes of global political and economic transformation under neoliberalism. These processes and relations transcend the productive and reproductive, the local and global, and serve to intimately connect individuals, households, NGOs, governments, international financial institutions, international organizations, and global development agencies.

ON METHODOLOGY

Empirically, this book examines the lived experiences and political practices of queer activists engaged in HIV prevention and other sexual rights work in Accra. It draws on extensive fieldwork carried out in Ghana between 2013 and 2014, including interviews with community activists, NGO activists, queer working-class men, and other allies, as well as participant observation and documentary analysis of media reports, policies, and other organizational materials.[17] The book aims to provide an in-depth account—a slice of "thick description"—of the key actors, forms of organizing, and political practices that constitute the first wave of queer activism in Accra, which emerged in the late 1990s and early 2000s.[18] This activism has been primarily linked to the HIV prevention and sexual rights activities of a small handful of NGOs that operate through what Cal Biruk calls the "the global health-human rights nexus" (2020:478), or what I term development's sexual health rights paradigm. The book brings together an ethnographer's concern for specificity—for the intimate, everyday, and embodied experiences of queer working-class men in Accra—with a political economist's concern for the structural and systematic, and for the interactions between macrolevel political economic systems and the microlevel dynamics of queer lives.

Participant observation is conventionally understood as the cornerstone of ethnographic research (Clifford and Marcus 1986). For the purposes of this study, I spent thirteen months engaged in participant observation at two Ghanaian NGOs, CEPEHRG and the Human Rights Advocacy Centre (HRAC), both of which are located in Accra, and among queer community networks. Accra is the administrative and economic capital of Ghana. It is a multilingual city with four main languages: Ga, the language of its native inhabitants, the Ga ethnic group; Akan, the cluster of dialects spoken by the country's largest and historically dominant ethnic group, the Akan;[19] Hausa, a Chadic language originating in northern Nigeria; and English, the language of Ghana's former colonial rulers, the British (Kropp Dakubu 1997).[20] Almost all the peer educators and community activists I met were multilingual, speaking at least one Ghanaian language in addition to English, and the majority of them came from either Ga or Akan ethnic backgrounds. Alongside English, Twi was the main language of communication used in the NGO offices, although both Twi and Ga were commonly spoken among staff. As part of my research, I learned to speak and write these two languages, Twi and Ga, achieving a basic level of proficiency.

In terms of participant observation, I spent several days a week at CEPEHRG and HRAC, observing day-to-day activities at the office and in the field, and the activities of the individuals who worked there. I also attended staff meetings, review sessions with CEPEHRG's network of peer educators, HIV testing and counselling programs, human rights sensitization workshops, values clarification sessions, and condom and lubricant distribution. Observations took place at different times, during working hours, in the evenings, and on weekends, in an attempt to capture different dimensions of life within the organization. In addition to my research at CEPEHRG and HRAC, over time I expanded my observations to include queer community networks across Accra. I focused my research in the geographic areas of central and coastal Accra: Jamestown, Bukom, Chorkor, Kokomlemle, and Adabraka. These areas were not identified according to a preestablished research design.[21] Rather, they were identified through the process of research itself, based on the relationships I had built with individuals living in these areas. As part of this, I attended birthday parties, funeral celebrations, engagement parties, weddings, and outdoorings, I went to Accra's queer-friendly bars, again largely in the Jamestown area, and I was invited to the homes of a number of queer acquaintances.[22]

ON LANGUAGE

The final section of this chapter sets out the structure of the book. Before that, I wish to clarify some of the key terms that will be used to describe sexual politics and activism in Ghana (and in Africa more generally).[23] Terminology in this regard is complex and contested. The acronym "LGBTI" (sometimes "LGBT" or "LGBT+") is commonly used in human rights and development spheres to designate a fixed set of sexual orientations and gendered identities—lesbian, gay, bisexual, trans, and intersex (Budhiraja, Fried, and Teixeira 2010). However, the extent to which the LGBTI identity model is applicable in Africa has been the subject of considerable debate (Matebeni 2014b; Nyanzi 2015; Tamale 2011). In her parody essay "How Not to Write about Queer South Africa," Zethu Matebeni begins by stating: "Always use the acronym LGBT in your writing. It sounds nice and it shows you are inclusive" (2014a:57).[24] Matebeni makes the point that the acronym has both a homogenizing and universalizing effect, especially when used by non-African writers: "In your text . . . they are all just gay," as she puts it.

Sylvia Tamale (2011:25) critiques the usage of LGBTI from a different angle, arguing that "the identity politics that underpin these Western notions do not necessarily apply in African contexts." Tamale's analysis goes beyond issues of cultural imperialism to raise a more fundamental, ontological question regarding the association of sexual practice with social identity, or the idea that one *is* gay, one *is* bisexual. Put otherwise, the practice-identity link implicit in LGBTI models is not compatible with the ways in which nonnormative sexual and gender relations are interpreted in different African settings and, more broadly, with culturally located understandings of personhood.[25] These various indigenous terms and idioms—which include *sasso* in Ghana, *kuchu* in Uganda, *matsoalle* in Lesotho, to name just a few—cannot be easily collapsed into, or enshrined within, fixed frameworks or categories. This book does not therefore use "LGBTI" to refer generically to individuals or groups in Ghana who diverge from heterosexual or cisgender norms. I do, however, use the LGBTI acronym to refer specifically to the ways in which this model of sexual orientation and gender identity circulates among human rights and development institutions and practitioners.

Responding, perhaps, to questions over the universal applicability of LGBTI identity models, the term "sexual minorities"—also "sexual and gender minorities"—has gained traction among some scholars of sexuality, health, and development (Corrêa, Petcheskey, and Parker 2008; Epprecht 2012; Gosine 2005; Jolly 2007; Park 2016). In Andrew Park's "A Development Agenda for Sexual Minorities" (2016:9), he defines sexual minorities using three core criteria: "1. People who describe themselves using sexual minority terminology. 2. People whose sexual partners are the same gender, or a minority gender. 3. People who experience attraction to individuals of the same or a minority gender." "Sexual minorities" in this articulation is intended to move away from static, identity-based models of gender and sexuality and to recognize that concepts of "sexual orientation" and "gender identity" are complex and multivalent. However, as Park's definition indicates, it is not always clarified within the literature whether minority is intended to denote minoritarian status—in terms of a lack of social, economic, or political power, or an absence of rights, for example—or to indicate a numerical minority. Whether intentional or not, I would argue that these numerical and normative connotations—that is, the implicit contrast with a sexual "majority"—risks abstracting gender and sexuality from their structural contexts and, in so doing, deracinating homophobia and oppression from power relations.

The relevance of queer theory to the study of sexualities in Africa has been similarly fraught with disagreement, including charges of "Westocentrism" (Epprecht 2013) and "western hegemony" (Nyanzi 2015). This debate shares some common ground with critiques of LGBTI identity models and politics, since the intellectual origins of queer theory are rooted in Europe and the United States. Queer theory is also understood to be enduringly associated with the work of Michel Foucault and Judith Butler and to have travelled beyond the Global North in ways that risk reproducing hegemonic (and non-African) ways of knowing (Nyanzi 2015). For Keguro Macharia (2016), the issue is not simply one of terminology—of LGBTI versus queer—or even about how queer theory travels "to" Africa. Rather, it is about epistemological power relations and the extractive ways in which research on African sexualities is used by Anglo-American academics. Thus, he argues (2016:185): "Queer African voices and experiences will be absorbed as 'data' or 'evidence,' not as modes of theory or as challenges to the conceptual assumptions that drive queer studies." Macharia's concerns recall the critiques of Western academic writing advanced by African feminist scholars discussed in the prologue (Oyěwùmí 1997; Tamale 2020), which emphasize the imperial footings of knowledge production about Africa in the West.

According to Stella Nyanzi (2015:61), the project of queering "Queer Africa" is therefore both empirical and epistemological in character: she writes, "One must simultaneously reclaim Africa in its bold diversities and reinsert queerness" and reject "western hegemony over queer studies" (2015:60). This argument is picked up by Rachel Spronk and Thomas Hendriks (2020:6), who call for an approach that studies sexualities *in* Africa *from* Africa (i.e., rather than producing studies *on* sexualities *in* Africa). This, they argue, is "a deceptively small lexicological difference that reflects a much broader epistemological and political stance." This stance is intended to use the productive tensions between queer theory and sexualities studies from Africa to reshape hegemonic ways of knowing about sex and gender at the global level. While I am not fully persuaded, given my positionality, that I can claim to be studying sexualities *from* Africa, this book aims to use African scholarship (and scholarship from across the diaspora) to think *with* and *through* African ways of knowing about non-normative sexualities. In so doing, I also seek to bring insights from this rich literature to bear on the study of global political economy.

Nyanzi's work contributes to a growing body of scholarship (Ekine and Abbas 2013; Matebeni et al. 2018; Matebeni and Pereira 2014; Nyanzi 2015) that employs and repurposes queer theoretical and methodological frameworks in order to study dissident sexual, gender, and body politics in the African context. This project of reclaiming and reframing queer theory is affirmed by Douglas Clarke, who argues that "Africa has a model for queer theory that is largely unexplored in the Western world" (2013:175). In conceptual terms, Zethu Matebeni and Jabu Pereira (2014:7) argue that queer is valuable in the African context because it creates "space that pushes the boundaries of what is embraced as normative." Similarly, Vasu Reddy et al. (2018) employ queer (and LGBTQ) as a means to challenge binaries, recognize diversity, and confront heteronormativity (while acknowledging the complexities and limitations of existing linguistic and conceptual frameworks). These formulations reiterate the centrality of "anti-normativity" to a queer theoretical approach, as articulated by key queer theorists such as David Halperin and Michael Warner.[26] Yet they also expand the conceptual boundaries of the anti-normative to better capture the realities of queer African lives and experiences, including how they are shaped by racism, white supremacy, and neocolonialism (and how heteronormativity is itself implicated within these structures). Matebeni (2017:26, italics mine) thus argues in favor of "reimagining the category queer not just as sexual or gender identity, but also as a form of *destabilizing notions of belonging attached to the racist and heteronormative neo-colonial project.*"[27]

As this suggests, the take-up of queer approaches in the study of African sexualities is important not only epistemologically and empirically, but also materially and politically, since it forms part of a transformative project intended to challenge sexual and gendered injustices in the status quo. In view of these contributions, this book draws on queer theory (and the terminology of "queer") in order to avoid eliding different, culturally specific configurations of gender and sexuality in Ghana and to trouble foundational assumptions regarding the links between biological sex, the body, gender, and sexual practice. Accordingly, my usage of "queer" is not intended to be read as an umbrella descriptor for sexual identities, as per the acronym "LGBTI," or as another identity category, as per the acronym "LGBTQ," which is how queer has come to circulate in some Anglo-American strains of identity politics and international human rights frames. In this identitiarian iteration, as David Eng and Jasbir Puar (2020:7) point out, "queer" is both productive and destructive of subjectivities, a "foil for the globalization of capital in its imperial travels." Instead, my usage of queer follows in the spirit of Matebeni's (2017) work: as anti-foundational and as a means to recognize the material bases of heteronormativity, as these are entwined in the histories and contemporalities of capitalism and (neo)colonialism. This is also consistent with a broader aim of this book: to outline an understanding of (queer) sexuality and gender as inherently "racial arrangements" under capitalism—to borrow C. Riley Snorton's phrase (2017)—and to consider how forms of sexual oppression and exploitation, in addition to those of race, gender, and class, are co-constitutive of, rather than epiphenomenal to, the global economy. This aim is indebted to a long-standing tradition of radical queer scholarship that shows why questions of "empire, race, migration, geography, subaltern communities, activism, and class" are central to the project of queer critique (Eng et al. 2005:2).

In the literature on Ghana, Otu's (2022) study of *sassoi*, self-identified effeminate men in southern Ghana, borrows the philosopher Kwame Gyekye's notion of "amphibious personhood" to describe *sasso*'s shifting subjective practices. These practices unsettle what Otu (2022) calls "Western categories of gender and sexuality" but are also consistent, in certain culturally located ways, with the queer refusal of identity. As Lee Edelman (2004: 17) notably argued, "Queerness can never define an identity; it can only ever disturb one." Otu thus clarifies his deployment of queer theory by reorienting the epistemological point of departure; in other words, he uses *sasso* subjectivities in Ghana to explore queerness, rather than queerness as a lens to explore *sasso* subjectivities. Elsewhere, Serena Dankwa, following in the tradition of Ruth Morgan and Saskia Wieringa in their work on intimate relations among women in Africa, eschews the terminology of queer to describe her Ghanaian research participants, whom, she notes, were frequently "unfamiliar or uncomfortable with terms like 'queer,' 'lesbian,' and 'bisexual'" (Dankwa 2021:15). Like Otu, Dankwa (2021) uses "queer" as an epistemological and theoretical tool, but favors indigenous interpretations that center intimacies and practices rather than "identities." She therefore uses the term "knowing women" to refer to her research participants.[28]

For the purposes of this book, I have chosen not to use the term *sasso* in a more generic way to refer to my research participants, despite its common circulation within working-class queer men's networks in southern Ghana. This is primarily because not all of my research participants used the term and indeed some explicitly rejected it as a descriptor. I acknowledge that, for some, my choice of "queer" as an alternative will be seen as imperfect, not least because the peer educators and community activists I met employed a wide-ranging lexicon of words and phrases to refer to their own sexual and gendered practices (among which queer rarely featured). In recognition of this limitation, where I refer to the subjective or naming practices of specific research participants, I aim to reproduce the language and terminology they used themselves.

Reflecting on the Ugandan context, Rahul Rao (2020:30) argues that the linguistic challenge of finding appropriate signifiers highlights the "inadequacies of both queer and *kuchu* as comprehensive placeholders for gender and sexual non-normativity." Rather, he suggests, scholars should be concerned with "the work such placeholders do" (Rao 2020:30). As well as encouraging us to think beyond the politics of naming, this argument recalls earlier queer scholarship that conceptualized "queer" as a verb and an action, as opposed to a noun: a "means of negotiating the complications" (Jakobsen 1998:515). According to Janet Jakobsen (1998:526), queer should not be defined in purely oppositional terms—that is, using a narrow interpretation of "antinormative"—but necessarily entails a move to resistance, agency, and, ultimately, solidarity (Jakobsen 1998:526).[29] This framing speaks to the broader feminist ethic behind this book, the transformative impulses underpinning the turn toward queer theory among scholars of African sexualities, and why queerness, as José Esteban Muñoz (2009:1) puts it, must insist on the "potentiality or concrete possibility for another world."

ORGANIZATION OF THE BOOK

This book is divided into five chapters.

Chapter 1: Toward a Political Economy of Queer Oppression and Resistance

This chapter sets out a political economy approach for studying queer oppression and resistance in Ghana. The chapter begins by surveying the existing literature on queer sexual politics in Africa, which I organize into three key frames, the "social movement," "queering development," and "globalization" frames. I put these frames into conversation with feminist and queer political economy scholarship in order to consider what they do (and, in a sense, do not) tell us about queer oppression and resistance in Ghana. Against this background, I set out the three core themes or "dimensions" of my political economy framework. These are, in brief, sexuality, capitalism, and the state; sexuality, capitalism, and global governance; and the everyday political economy of queer lives and resistance. In the second half of the chapter, I begin to parse how this framework illuminates the landscape of queer sexual politics in Ghana, with a particular focus on historicizing homophobia through the colonial and postcolonial state.

Chapter 2: The NGO-ization of Queer Activism in Ghana

This chapter troubles genealogies of queer African activism that take the HIV epidemic as the sole or primary point of departure, based on a case study of CEPEHRG, Ghana's first and most prominent LGBTI/HIV organization. The chapter begins by setting out the broader shifts in development and global health policy that have shaped the field of queer Ghanaian politics over the past fifteen years, namely the growing currency of concepts of "sexual rights," increasing recognition of sexual orientation and gender identity and LGBTI rights as "development issues," and the move toward a "key population" paradigm in national Ghanaian HIV policy. It shows how these shifts have both informed and transformed first-wave activists' approaches to LGBTI rights. The chapter then outlines some of the key modes of organizing, political practices, and types of action adopted by CEPEHRG, showing how processes of NGOization have shaped the organization's trajectory. I conclude the chapter by highlighting the impact of politicized homophobia—both institutional and everyday—and activists' personal experiences of violence and oppression on formal queer activism and understandings of LGBTI rights. These experiences shed light on the contradictory and at times regressive impacts of development interventions on the field of queer Ghanaian politics, as well as activists' struggles to advance queer struggle in the face of politicized homophobia.

Chapter 3: HIV Prevention, Peer Education, and Queer Labor in the Global Development Industry

This chapter examines claims that development interventions on sexual health rights are "empowering" for queer African communities. Building on the case study of CEPEHRG set out in Chapter 2, it shows how emerging forms of queer resistance in Ghana have not only been co-opted into but divided by the structures and power relations of the global development industry, focusing in particular on queer men's work in peer education. The chapter begins with the story of Adam, a former peer educator and community activist who has given up on NGO-ized spheres of queer politics in Ghana. Theoretically, the chapter reads peer education through the lens of social reproduction, that is, as a modality of unpaid caring labor that is systematically devalued and frequently invisibilized in the global economy. The chapter further shows how, contrary to its "empowerment" aims, peer education programs fuel and reinforce the divide between formal and informal strands of queer activism in Ghana—between the more middle-class spheres of civil society and the working-class queer networks of Accra—and place a disproportionate burden of responsibility for tackling the HIV epidemic on queer working-class men. The chapter contextualizes these dynamics in relation to the emergence of a neoliberal empowerment paradigm in global development discourse, as well as wider shifts in the organization of social reproduction across the Global South.

Chapter 4: Queer Ghanaian Politics beyond Sexual Health

This chapter sets out the priorities and practices of queer struggle in Ghana beyond the purview of development and NGO-led sexual health rights work. It begins by elucidating how HIV narratives of "behavior change" interact with experiences of homophobia, shaping activists' understanding of their own embodied practices and, ultimately, reinforcing heterosexist norms. I analyze this in relation to widespread anti-queer violence in Ghana and highlight the regressive consequences of selective health-oriented approaches to LGBTI rights from an embodied and ideational perspective. The chapter goes on to delineate four key priorities for queer struggle as identified through the narrative testimonies and everyday practices of queer community activists in Accra: ending homophobic violence; addressing poverty and raising standards of living; finding decent work; and improving mental health and well-being. In the second part of the chapter, I examine how queer community activists and groups are resisting and pushing back against homophobia and oppression at a grassroots level, on the issues that are important to them. They do so through four primary activities: queer kinship practices, claiming and queering space, community mediation, and legal rights claims. These practices and modes of organizing address, on their own terms and in their own ways, the priorities for struggle identified above.

Conclusion: The Current and Future Frontiers of Queer African Activism

The concluding chapter of this book takes a big-picture look at the current and future frontiers of queer struggle in Africa and beyond. It begins by highlighting organizing around decriminalization in Botswana, Kenya, and a number of other African states, and reflects on the strategic importance of decriminalization in the Ghanaian context. Following this, the chapter reads the vision for queer liberation set out in the 2010 African LGBTI manifesto alongside the political priorities of queer community activists in Ghana and considers what this means for a liberatory and transnational queer politics, beyond a Global North / Global South binary. Against this background, I summarize the core findings of this book—namely, that sexual health rights approaches are inadequate to address the materiality of queer oppression in Ghana and therefore the multiplicity of struggle—and highlight the implications of these findings for scholars, activists, and policymakers invested in tackling sexual injustice and oppression around the world.

CHAPTER 1

Toward a Political Economy of Queer Oppression and Resistance

The economic, tied to the reproductive, is necessarily linked to the reproduction of heterosexuality. It is not that non-heterosexual forms of sexuality are simply left out, but that their suppression is essential to the operation of that prior normativity.
—Judith Butler, "Merely Cultural" (1998:42)

To observe that the genealogy of modern liberalism is simultaneously a genealogy of colonial divisions of humanity is a project of tracking the ways in which race, geography, nation, caste, religion, gender, sexuality and other social differences become elaborated as normative categories for governance under the rubrics of liberty and sovereignty.
—Lisa Lowe, *The Intimacies of Four Continents* (2015:7)

INTRODUCTION: QUEER SOCIAL MOVEMENTS IN AFRICA

In the academic literature, a substantive body of empirical research on queer activism in Africa did not start to emerge until the 2000s, especially on contexts beyond South Africa. Ashley Currier's scholarship (2010, 2012, 2015, 2016, 2018) has made an important contribution to the field by examining LGBTI movement politics across parts of southern Africa and Malawi. Using the lens of social movement theory, this work centralizes the political constraints and opportunities shaping formal activism in different country contexts and explores the strategic implications for movement dynamics, both nationally and internationally. In her book *Politicizing Sex in Contemporary Africa*, Currier (2018) connects this long-standing interest in movement dynamics to the analysis of "politicized homophobia" in Malawi. According to Currier (2018:1), politicized homophobia is "a strategy used by African political elites interested in consolidating their moral and political authority." At the level of activism in Malawi, politicized homophobia has divided civil society, "undermining solidarity partnerships between NGOs" (Currier 2018:43). This analysis deftly illuminates how homophobia is being mobilized by some political elites as a strategy and mechanism of state control and how this is relational to (i.e., rather than independent from) the activities of activists and other civil society actors.

In the West African context, Patrick Awondo (2010) similarly uses the lens of social movement theory to examine the emergence of two "homosexual organizations" in Cameroon, Association de Défense des Homosexuels and Alternatives Cameroun, which focus on sexual rights and sexual health respectively. These organizations have been both enabled and constrained by their engagements with global development organizations, national institutions, and human rights frameworks, a set of interactions that have also impacted on their strategic development. In essence, Awondo finds that external support may be pragmatically appealing in the short term for LGBTI organizations in contexts like Cameroon, in terms of access to resources. But it may also lead to "delegitimization . . . in places formerly under colonial rule, where homosexuality has become a part of the cause of cultural nationalism" (Awondo 2010:326).

There are certainly parallels between Currier's and Awondo's findings in Malawi and Cameroon and the Ghanaian case, where, from the outset, the founders of CEPEHRG, Ghana's first formal LGBTI/HIV organization, ran into difficulties in setting up and sustaining a "visible" advocacy group. According to CEPEHRG's executive director, Evans-Love Quansah, one key challenge was funding. Another challenge was the hostile political climate surrounding the issue of LGBTI rights, which included opposition from some sections of Ghanaian civil society. Like Charles Yeboah, Evans emphasizes that CEPEHRG's work on LGBTI rights has been too isolated and inconsistent to be viewed as belonging to any kind of social movement. As historically the only formal organization in Ghana to explicitly work on LGBTI rights at the community level, Evans's reticence on the subject of movement-building is understandable. CEPEHRG's relative isolation within the field of Ghanaian civil society has been compounded by the geopolitics of aid funding, which has tended to prioritize funding for HIV prevention rather than support for LGBTI activism in Africa (Wallace et al. 2018). These dynamics, as I show in Chapter 2, have decisively shaped the organization's political and organizational trajectory.

According to Epprecht (2013:168), the strategy of shrouding LGBTI rights in the more "neutral" language of sexual health has proved strategically beneficial for some grassroots movement organizations in Africa, especially in regions outside of southern Africa, where openly advocating for LGBTI rights may entail significant political and personal risk. However, in the Ghanaian context, development-funded activities on HIV have also played a key part in driving the politicization of homosexuality, not least by rendering MSM visible in new and contradictory ways. These dynamics are starkly illuminated by the media frenzy over the "registration" of homosexuals in the Western and Central Regions of Ghana in 2006, discussed in the prologue, which brought together a powerful set of anxieties over HIV, sexually transmitted "diseases," and homosexuality. Put otherwise, sexual health approaches that frame MSM rights primarily in epidemiological terms can be highly politicizing in and of themselves, since they position MSM as both bearers of rights and threats to public health. The complex, multiscalar interactions between sexual rights paradigms, HIV prevention initiatives, and politicized homophobia in Ghana are explored in detail in Chapters 3 and 4 of this book.

In terms of social movement theory, the case of CEPEHRG suggests that examining how movement dynamics shape formal strands of LGBTI organizing in Ghana can yield some insights, but that this approach may not be appropriate to capture the shifting and contingent character of queer networks and organizing and how this relates to the HIV epidemic and the politicization of homosexuality. Methodologically, a social movement framing also seems less suitable in the Ghanaian case, in light of both the warnings of Evans and Charles and the relatively limited number of formal movement organizations involved in the first wave of queer activism—essentially one grassroots organization, a small number of predominantly sexual health-focused groups with overlapping interests in MSM rights, and one larger human rights organization that prioritizes "minority rights." Nonetheless, the social movement literature's analytical focus on the state as a key actor in mobilizing and instrumentalizing politicized homophobia is instructive. I bring this focus together with insights from feminist and queer political economy to inform the first dimension in my theoretical framework, which I conceptualize as the role of the (capitalist) state in producing and regulating sexualities.

SEXUALITY, CAPITALISM, AND THE STATE

As Suzanne Bergeron and Jyoti Puri (2012: 493) highlight, the state is a particularly "dense node of governance" when it comes to sexuality. State laws, policies, and practices shape the lives of queer populations in myriad ways, most obviously through criminalization, but also through exclusion from employment, citizenship, and the right to family life; the denial of health care and other basic services; and restrictions on freedom of expression, association, and assembly.[1] At a structural level, the state is important both in terms of its impact on queer populations and as a sexualized and gendered construct; that is, the state produces and is produced by sexuality (Puri 2016). One example of this is the production and reification of the gender binary through early Western state-making practices: "Making states makes sex," as V. Spike Peterson puts it (2014b:390). Peterson's work shows how binary sex and gender (i.e., male-female sex and masculine-female gender identities) were codified and institutionalized through laws concerning marriage, tax, inheritance, property, and citizenship and through the constitution of differently gendered socioeconomic spheres. These laws structured social reproduction—for example, through the regulation of reproductive sexual activities—and the transmission of property and citizenship along heteropatriarchal and racialized lines. This, in turn, ensured the continuance of particular Western state formations over time (Peterson 2014a:605; see also Chitty 2020).

While Peterson's (2014b) genealogy goes back as far as the Greek city-states, for the purpose of this analysis, the transition to capitalism provides a more fruitful point of departure for grasping the gendered, racialized, and sexualized character of state laws and governance practices. As Silvia Federici (2004) documents, from the mid-sixteenth century onwards, state laws in Europe reinforced processes of primitive accumulation and dispossession by institutionalizing particular types of patriarchal property, household, and labor relations. Federici focuses in particular on the enclosures, which, she argues, entailed and accompanied new forms of gendered violence and coercion. This included the introduction of laws that prohibited contraception, abortion, and infanticide, as part of a broader set of changes that effectively removed women's control over reproduction. It is in this context that "a new sexual division of labor" was forged, whereby women's bodies were increasingly subordinated, confined to the domestic, family sphere, and used as "instruments" for the reproduction of the workforce (Federici 2004:100). Taken together, these shifts worked to shape and shore up an emergent (proto)capitalist economic order.

Primitive accumulation was dependent not only on the control of gendered and sexualized bodies and labor in the "core," however, but on the violent exploitation of racialized bodies and labor in the colonial "peripheries" (Federici 2004; see also Drucker 2015; Sears 2017). The transition to capitalism thus enmeshed sexuality and the body within capitalist social relations and processes of class formation, *and* within the projects of imperial conquest and slavery. In so doing, it established a new role (and set of incentives) for the state, both domestically and in the colonial territories, in the control and regulation of sexual and body politics.

By the nineteenth century, the interrelationship of empire, capitalist development, racial oppression, and patriarchal subjugation had been both consolidated and further transformed (McClintock 1995; Stoler 2002). During this period, gender and sexual norms in Europe were increasingly restricted and disciplined through an expanding state apparatus of laws, institutions, and governance practices linked to both industrialization and (high) imperial expansion (Drucker 2015). This apparatus, which included intensified legal restrictions on prostitution and sexual relations between men, worked to uphold specifically heteronormative configurations of sexuality, gender, and family (heterosexual, married, procreative, cisgender, binary, nuclear, etc.) and to posit a binary between the (normal) heterosexual and the (abject) homosexual. Thus, as Rosemary Hennessy (2000:97) notes, "Western industrialized societies' heteronormative sexual identity and its perverse others gradually coalesce at about the same time commodity culture does—at the height of nineteenth-century imperialism."

Rather than transporting norms of gender and sexuality to their colonies, European imperial powers solidified ideals of (middle class, white) womanhood through their discursive opposition to the "savage" and "backward" sexuality of colonized populations, especially in Africa (McClintock 1995; Stoler 2002). In this way, the construction of normative sexuality in the nineteenth century was discursively grounded in (liberal) ideas of "modernity" and "civility" and materially enacted through prohibitive legal frameworks backed up by regimes of gendered, sexualized, racialized, and class-based violence. As McClintock (1995:5) argues, "Imperialism and the invention of race were fundamental aspects of Western, industrial modernity . . . central not only to the self-definition of the middle class but also to the policing of the 'dangerous classes': the working class, the Irish, Jews, prostitutes, feminists, gays and lesbians, criminals, the militant crowd and so on." This reveals the key disciplinary role of sexual and gender norms in the era of industrial modernity and how normative disciplinary power was produced through the subjugation and sanctioning of the non-normative (Foucault 1978; Butler 1998; see also Smith 2020). It also illuminates why emergent structures of heteronormativity were not only historically contingent and linked to shifts in the social relations of (re)production, but always already racialized in character (Ferguson 2004; see also Davis 1981; Spillers 1987; Snorton 2017).

As this brief overview suggests, any genealogy of the "sexual state," to borrow Puri's term (2016), in Ghana must be interwoven with the history of "colonial capitalism" (Ince 2018).[2] Colonial rule in what was then the "Gold Coast" established new systems and laws governing land, property, and labor (based on capitalism) and new religious, political, and education systems and institutions (based on Christianity, liberalism, and European education models respectively) (Tamale 2020:6). These shifts necessitated the transformation and production of gender and sexual relations and norms. Exploring these dynamics in the Yoruban context, Oyèrónkẹ́ Oyěwùmí (1997:31) shows that gender was not "an organizing principle in Yoruba society prior to colonization by the West." Rather, precolonial Yoruba society was socially organized by seniority, defined by relative age. This system was reconfigured during the colonial era, notably through the construction of "men" and "women" as concrete and binary social categories (see also Amadiume 1987). These changes worked to establish what Maria Lugones (2007:190) calls the "colonial/modern gender system," which was premised on sexual dimorphism, patriarchy, and heterosexuality (i.e., heteronormativity), as well as racial hierarchies.

Heteronormativity can be defined as "the institutions, structures of understanding, and practical orientations that make heterosexuality seem not only coherent—that is, organized as a sexuality—but also privileged" (Berlant and Warner 1998:548). It refers to the vast web of political, legal, social, and economic norms and practices that delimit what forms sex and gender can take and render these forms coherent and cohesive. Heteronormativity thus works across micro, meso, and macro scales, through the site of the (patriarchal) family/household, state practices and laws, structures of global governance, and "sexualized orders of international relation" (Weber 2016:6). It is further tied to temporally and spatially differentiated relations of production and social reproduction. In the contemporary Ghanaian context, heteronormativity is (re)produced through the state, the legal system—including laws relating to marriage, tax, inheritance, and property—the education system, religious institutions, and family and household arrangements, which include the gender division of labor. It is also enacted through an array of everyday social practices relating to gender and sexuality, from the way people dress to the norms that govern dating, sex, and relationships.[3] While the origins of many of these laws and norms trace back to the colonial era, they were also reshaped by sweeping macroeconomic changes in the decades following independence. I explore some of these dynamics in the final section of this chapter.

SEXUALITY, POLITICIZED HOMOPHOBIA, AND THE (POSTCOLONIAL) STATE

So far, this analysis has illuminated the key regulatory and coercive powers of the state vis-à-vis intimate and family relations (both historically and contemporarily), what is at stake in these relations in political economic terms (and in specific relation to processes of accumulation and dispossession), and how injustices arising from heteronormativity produce, and are produced by, other class-based, gendered, racialized, and territorialized injustices.[4] I propose this account of sexuality and the state as a metaframe for the more fine-grained analysis of how struggles over citizenship, sovereignty, and national identity come to be played out on the terrain of sexuality in contexts of postcoloniality, as part of "state nationalism and its sexualization of particular bodies" (Alexander 1994:6). Again, these struggles have *consequences* for queer populations, in terms of engendering certain types of sexual oppression and injustice, and work to shape and *constitute* queer subjectivities and relations, by positioning them in opposition to the norm. As Basile Ndjio argues, in many postcolonial African countries, the "nationalization" of sexuality has enabled the state to construct new modes of (sexual) citizenship, which demarcate the boundaries between "Africans and Westerners, citizens and strangers, authentic and deracinated Africans, good and bad citizens, loyal and disloyal subjects" (2013:128).

Uganda is one such example, where "homophobic nationalism" has been tied to, and articulated through, a state project of sexual citizenship. This project aims to shore up state legitimacy and functionality and to promote national unity, namely by galvanizing public opinion against a common enemy: homosexuality (Rodriguez 2017:397). While the Ghanaian government had, up until recently, pursued a less hardline position on homosexuality than their Ugandan counterparts, the politicization of homosexuality since the early 2000s has similarly worked to imbricate homophobia within political narratives that seek to carve out a Ghanaian national identity, as well as postcolonial struggles over sovereignty and anti-imperialism. In this context, nationalism constitutes a key component in the political mobilization of homophobia in Ghana. In this book, however, I adopt Currier's (2018) concept of "politicized homophobia" to describe this trajectory because it captures the processual, relational, and agentive character of homophobia as it has been deployed strategically by Ghanaian political elites (see also Tettey 2016). As Currier (2018:1) explains: "This strategy necessitates that elites activate and politicize homophobia; the act of politicization turns homophobia from an interpersonal phenomenon into a wider set of anti-homosexual discourses and practices that saturate political rhetoric." Viewed through this lens, moments of moral panics, such as those that occurred in 2006 and 2011, are key parts of the "act of politicization."

I would add that understandings of politicized homophobia and the nationalization of sexuality can be sharpened by considering how homophobia as a state strategy relates to broader dynamics of capitalist crisis and how, therefore, the cultural and political production of panic is enmeshed with the economic. I am drawing on the work of the sociologist Stuart Hall (1978) here, who sets out a specific explanation of "moral panic" that is rooted in the material politics of capitalist crisis and state response:

> When the official reaction to a person, groups of persons or series of events is out of all proportion to the actual threat offered, when "experts," in the form of Police chiefs, the judiciary, politicians and editors perceive the threat in all but identical terms, and appear to talk "with one voice" of rates, diagnoses, prognoses and solutions, when the media representations universally stress sudden and dramatic increases (in numbers involved or events) and "novelty," above and beyond that which a sober, realistic appraisal could sustain, then we believe it is appropriate to speak of the beginnings of a moral panic. (Hall 1978:16)

Although Hall was writing about a very different political context (1970s Britain), phenomenon (mugging), and set of economic crisis conditions (stagflation), his description of moral panic could easily apply to the contemporary Ghanaian context (with, perhaps, the addition of religious leaders to the list of "experts").[5] Hall's framing invites us to think of moral panics as never exclusively or essentially "moral" in character. Rather, they are bound up in political economy, in how states exercise power through mechanisms such as the law and the police, but also through the field of everyday culture, such as the media.[6] As Rao (2020:163) notes: "The precarity of everyday life under neoliberalism has exacerbated popular anxieties. . . . Moral panics thrive in the fertile soil of these anxieties, fastening on a range of marginal figures including queers, sex workers, 'witches,' women who wear short skirts, and others who appear to disrupt normative kinship." Thus, the figure of the "homosexual"—deviant, pathological, unnatural, un-African—serves to legitimate increasingly authoritarian political interventions, including expanded criminalization. These acts of politicization are a way of "policing the crisis" (Hall 1978) that divert attention away from deep-seated problems of political economy: poverty, unemployment, precarity, inequality.

SEXUALITY IN/AND DEVELOPMENT

Whereas the social movement scholarship usefully sheds light on the role of the state and politicized homophobia in shaping the opportunities and constraints facing queer activists in Africa, the "queering development" literature centralizes the role of supra-state (and sub-state) governance and development processes in transforming intimate relations across the Global South (Jolly 2000, 2007; Lind 2009, 2010; Budhijira, Fried, and Teixeira 2010). Queering development challenges the assumption that development has historically ignored matters of sexuality. From population control programs to disease prevention initiatives, "the development industry has always dealt with sexuality-related issues" (Jolly 2010:23), albeit by framing sexuality primarily in terms of reproductive sex, disease, risk, and danger (Gosine 2005; Jolly 2010).

Not unlike state practices, the disciplinary and regulatory effects of global development policy and practice on intimate relations are bound up in both heteronormativity and capitalist political economy. Across key policy areas such as gender equality and poverty reduction, development has promoted a heterosexual "two-partner model of love and labour" (Bedford 2005:301) linked to Western ideals of the nuclear family (Drucker 2009) and excluded other non-normative household arrangements (Bergeron 2010). This draws attention to who is left out of global development interventions—namely queer and transgender people, and other queer configurations of love, desire, kinship, family, and corporeality—and the economic power relations and processes these exclusions serve to advance, namely market-based models of economic growth.

More recently, however, development institutions have moved to include LGBTI rights and LGBTI populations within development paradigms, notably through the adoption of pro-LGBTI politics within international financial institutions (IFIs) such as the World Bank (Bedford 2009; Rao 2015). According to Rao (2015:47), this forms part of a discursive strategy to fold certain "sanitized" queers into the project of neoliberal global capitalism. Drawing on Puar's (2013) work, IFIs' emerging support for LGBTI rights is understood as a homonormative and "homonationalist" project that conceals the political economic structures underpinning homophobia and sexual injustice around the world and the active role of IFIs in (re)producing these relations. In Puar's (2013:336) influential articulation, homonationalism describes how LGBTI rights have become "a barometer by which the right to and capacity for national sovereignty is evaluated." By categorizing nation-states into "gay friendly" or "homophobic," homonationalist discourse constructs new (racialized, neocolonial) dividing lines between the "civilized" and the "savage" worlds (Puar 2013:337). Within development policy and practice, this is articulated through a broader politics of "rescue," whereby gays have replaced women—and gay rights have supplanted women's rights—as the Global North's preferred barometer of modernity, civilization, and sovereignty in the Global South (Rao 2015; Puar 2007). Against this background, David Cameron's comments about the status of LGBTI rights in Ghana reflects the homonationalist ways in which racialized queer populations are invoked by Western leaders and thus how the politicization of homosexuality is, to borrow Rao's (2020) framing, transnationally produced.[7]

Turning to development interventions on HIV and sexual rights, Andil Gosine (2013:477) argues that "the particular ways in which MSM have been brought into the fold as targets and clients of development have come at an enormous cost," primarily because MSM are framed as a public health risk to heterosexual populations. While Gosine focuses on the Caribbean, there are similarities with Ghana, where efforts to address HIV amongst MSM, including by collecting better epidemiological data, have contributed to, and dovetailed with, the politicization of homosexuality. One effect of this, as noted earlier, has been to bolster homophobic stereotypes that view gay men as "vectors" of disease; another effect has been to generate biomedical data on a stigmatized population that can be manipulated and misinterpreted by homophobic political and media actors to stir up panic, as occurred in 2011 (Gyamerah 2021). I build on these insights in Chapter 3 by analyzing the implications of MSM peer education programs in relation to the politicization of homosexuality in Ghana and a broader neoliberal empowerment paradigm in global development discourse. I argue that this paradigm has rationalized the mobilization and exploitation of queer men's voluntary and unpaid caring labor, as a key strategy of HIV response.

In sum, queering development reveals how development institutions, policies, and practices may serve to reinforce structures and relations of hetero- and homonormativity, across different sites and scales (beyond the nation-state). These relations are, moreover, essentially compatible with neoliberal, market-led models of economic growth (Drucker 2009; Lind 2010). Rather than adopting a state-centric approach, this lens centralizes the "*layers of institutions* that are involved in defining and regulating our intimate lives" (Lind 2009:35, italics mine), which includes inter- and supranational organisations, IFIs, development agencies, and NGOs. It also illuminates why the political economy of development matters for understanding queer politics in Africa, particularly in terms of the regulatory and disciplinary power of development interventions and how this connects to hegemonic models of economic development. Vice versa, queer sexual politics matter for the global development industry because of the relationship between particular household/family models and neoliberal imperatives of growth, between normative configurations of sexuality and gender and the geopolitics of citizenship and nationhood, and between intimate relations and key areas of development policy, such as health, gender equality, education, and poverty reduction. These insights inform the second dimension in my political economy framework, which I conceptualize as the relationship between capitalism, sexuality, and global governance.

SEXUALITY IN/AND GLOBALIZATION

Interest in evolving modes of global governance and queer politics ties into a long-standing concern among scholars of sexuality and political economy: on the impact of globalization on sexual subjectivities, lifestyles, and patterns

of consumption (Altman 1996; Hennessy 2000, Drucker 2015). This literature highlights the role of globalization in giving rise to gay consumer cultures across parts of the Global South (Altman 1996, 1997; see also Hennessey
2000), as well as the establishment of transnational industries that capitalize
on Westerners' "imperial desires," through (white) gay international tourism,
NGOs, and volunteering (Alexander 2005; see also Hennessy 2000; Puar
2002; Meiu 2017).[8] According to Dennis Altman, "Economic and cultural globalization is creating a newly universal sense of homosexuality as the basis
for identity and lifestyle, not merely for behaviour" (1996:6). This forms part
of a wider process of "global queering" (Altman 1996), sometimes also called
the "universalization" of gay rights (Massad 2007) or "queer globalization"
(Binnie 2004).

Altman's claim that globalization has entailed the universalization of
Western sexual identities (and thus the homogenization of local queer cultures) has proved contentious (Tellis and Bala 2015), with research from Latin
America (Wright 2000; Lind and Share 2010), Southeast Asia (Boellstorff
2005, 2007, 2012; Jackson 2000), the Caribbean (Wekker 2006), and southern Africa (Hoad 2007), inter alia, emphasizing both similitude and difference in the translocation of LGBTI identities. This evidence unsettles the idea
of "hegemony from core to periphery" (Wright 2000:107) and reveals how
grassroots actors navigate global influences, Western identity models, and
unequal power relations in context-specific ways. This includes using funding
aimed at tackling HIV to establish and formalize domestic LGBTI movement
organizations and reformulating identity-based claims in order to advance
local queer political agendas (Lind and Share 2010; khanna 2009). While
development's "obsession with bad sex" (Jolly 2010) has been critiqued for its
symbolic and material implications, the sexual rights agenda (and the funding attached to it) has also been repurposed by activists in different country
contexts in ways that reflect both structure and agency. This is why, according to Neville Hoad, "The cultural imperialism model needs to be nuanced
by acknowledging that ideas, strategies, and identities are transformed when
they are used from below" (2007:35–36).

The literature on sexuality and globalization throws into relief the varie-
gated ways in which (queer) globalization has played out across the Global
South, how these dynamics are linked to patterns of uneven development,
and what this means for queer identities and activism across different settings. This brings to mind John D'Emilio's (1993) early work on capitalism
and sexuality, which argued that the emergence of gay identity in Europe and

North America was entwined in the rise of industrial capitalism and system of wage labor. These shifts divested the household of its functions as an independent economic unit and, combined with changing social mores during the early twentieth century (notably the separation of sex from procreation), enabled some urban men and women to increasingly organize their lives around queer sexual desires and relationships. In essence, capitalism—here linked to processes of proletarianization and urbanization—created the material conditions in which gay and lesbian communities were made possible and, by the 1970s, for the establishment of sexual identity as the basis for political organizing.

Given its Euro-American focus, D'Emilio's trajectory is not directly applicable to Ghana, where capitalist accumulation is not reducible to industrialization, where a (predominantly informal) urban proletariat continues to coexist with "a rural (and peri-urban) peasant subsistence realm" (Ossome 2021:71; Naidu and Ossome 2016), and where sexual and gender norms have been shaped and transformed through centuries of colonial encounter (i.e., not just during the economic and social upheaval of the nineteenth century). From a theoretical perspective, however, this line of analysis usefully illuminates how changing material conditions associated with capitalist transformation—shifts in the nature of work, the structure of labor markets, income levels, standards of living, dominant household arrangements, and the organization of social reproduction—may enable and produce certain affective and/or erotic ties and ways of being, including sexual identities and practices (see also Hennessy 2000; Drucker 2015). In Ghana, the decoupling of the family unit from production has been more partial than in Europe and North America, and marriage and biological reproduction remain highly valued, for both men and women (Clark 1999; Adomako Ampofo et al. 2009). Even in an urban context, where there has been a shift toward more nuclear models of family since the 1980s, the extended family form continues to hold power (Agyemang et al. 2018). This means that heteronormativity works through a range of family and household arrangements in the contemporary Ghanaian state, as well as constructs of femininity and masculinity. Moreover, this web of norms and (gendered and sexualized) power relations has material as well as cultural bases.

At the same time, globalization has profoundly reshaped the landscape of queer sexual politics in Ghana. One key aspect of this, as this chapter has highlighted, is the politicization of homosexuality, which has served to bring queer populations into the purview of the state and other governance actors in ways that are both unprecedented and rooted in Ghana's specific sexual history. Hoad sheds light on this complex of new and old in the South African context by analyzing globalization, decolonization, and colonialism as inter-connected processes shaping the politics of homosexuality (Hoad 2007:xvi). Drawing on Achille Mbembe's concept of the "subjective economy," he notes that contemporary sexual politics in South Africa are "underpinned by the economy of centuries of imperial material interest in this part of the world" (Hoad 2007: xvi). This underscores the importance of connecting (new) cultural-ideological and religious dynamics—such as the rise of homopho-bic rhetoric among prominent political and religious leaders—to historic and contemporary political processes and phenomena: colonization, the inde-pendence struggle, projects of postcolonial statebuilding, neoliberal devel-opment processes, the HIV epidemic. It also demonstrates why grounded empirical studies of queer sexual politics in Africa and across other parts of the Global South are needed, in order to understand "what globalization actually looks like from the perspective of working-class people who are liv-ing it" (Wekker 2006:224) and, I would add, how this is shaped by the after-lives of colonialism.

These distinct but overlapping literatures—what I have termed the "social movement," "queering development," and "globalization" literatures—raise important, interconnected questions about the role of the state in shaping queer sexual politics, the material resources and constraints that delimit formal modes of queer activism in Africa, the assimilation of queer sexual-ity into global health and sexual rights paradigms within development pol-icy and practice, and the unequal power relations, economic interests, and political agendas that inhere in development interventions in Africa. These are all questions that I seek to address, in some way, in this book. To do so, I have sought to fuse together and advance these insights by formulat-ing a political economy framework through which to study queer oppres-sion and resistance. This framework is intended to facilitate the analysis of activism in Ghana and in other parts of the world, especially in countries in the Global South marked by colonialism.[9] While the first dimension of the framework centers the role of capitalism and the state in producing and regulating sexualities, the second dimension centers the relationship between capitalism, sexuality, and global governance (specifically for this book, global development policies and practices relating to HIV and sexual rights). In addition to this, the third and final dimension aims to grapple with questions of structure, agency, and resistance in the context of global political economic change; I conceptualize this as a concern for the everyday political economies of queer lives and resistance.

SEXUALITY AND THE POLITICAL ECONOMY OF THE EVERYDAY

Scholars have identified a turn to the "everyday" in feminist studies of international political economy (Elias and Roberts 2016, Elias and Rethel 2018). This builds on a diverse and established tradition of feminist political economy scholarship that documents the gendered character of global economic processes and their implications for women's everyday productive and reproductive lives. This kind of political economy understands seemingly separate systems of oppression—gender, race, sexuality—as structurally related to, and therefore as structural features of, the global capitalist economy (Davis 1981; Petersen 2003; McNally 2017; Bhattacharya 2017). "Feminist political economies of the everyday" (Elias and Roberts 2016:3) examine how these co-constitutive relations play out at the level of the *everyday*, through the intimate, the embodied, and the mundane. By centralizing the activities and practices of ordinary people—and of socially and/or geographically marginalized groups—everyday political economy promises to reverse the line of inquiry from top down to bottom up and, in so doing, to illuminate how local actors shape, and are shaped by, the global economy. The point here is not simply that the global affects the local, the macro affects the micro, but that non-elite and, importantly, non-Western actors' engagements with, and articulations of, everyday political economic processes may both reproduce and resist broader patterns of global economic change. While studies of everyday political economy can take various forms—from studies of the household under neoliberalism (LeBaron 2010), to bingo regulation (Bedford 2016) and the global banana industry (Enloe 2000)—in this book, it is queer men's engagement with global development programs and actors, their embodied experiences of development work and activism, and how this connects to what Juanita Elias and Adrienne Roberts (2016:787) term "localized forms of resistance" that I focus on.

My concern for the political economy of the everyday also resonates with calls for scholars of queer African sexualities to understand lived experience in all its breadth and complexity, including in terms of "relationships, pleasure, intimacy, parenthood, education, voice and expression, representation and visibility, housing and shelter, movement, migration, exile and asylum, employment, income generation, livelihoods, family, ritual, health, spirituality, religion, faith, violence, security and safety, nationalism, ethnicity, and globalization" (Nyanzi 2014:63; see also Spronk and Nyeck 2021). Thus, while my framework posits sexuality in/and the state and global governance as key analytical dimensions for the study of queer oppression and resistance, this final dimension aims to encompass more quotidian microlevel practices, formations, and power relations (i.e., in addition to the state and suprastate levels), as well as the acts and forms of resistance that challenge them (i.e., in addition to mainstream social movements). In so doing, it seeks to advance what S. N. Nyeck (2021:2) calls the "non-standardized examination of everyday life as a practice of queer agency and theorizing."

To summarize, the political economy framework set out in this chapter provides three core dimensions through which to study queer oppression and resistance in Ghana and, I hope, in other parts of the global economy. While these dimensions are overlapping and interconnected rather than discrete, for the purposes of clarity I have sought to structure the book in a way that broadly addresses each dimension in turn. The first dimension is therefore primarily examined in the remainder of this chapter (and has already been partially explored in the introduction), the second dimension in Chapters 2 and 3, and the third dimension in Chapters 4 and the conclusion. Before turning to my case study of CEPEHRG, the final section of this chapter expands on the role of the state in producing and disciplining queer sexualities in Ghana. I do so in light of contemporary developments such as the politicization of homosexuality and by historicizing the governance of non-normative sexualities in Ghana in relation to the colonial and postcolonial state.

HISTORICIZING HOMOPHOBIA IN GHANA

From the imposition of laws criminalizing homosexual relations across Britain's colonies to the brutalities enacted on Two-Spirit people through settler-colonialism (Driskill 2004; Morgensen 2011), imperial incursions into gender and sexuality have always involved heteronormativity's "Others." The role of colonialism in establishing the legal, institutional, and cultural contexts in which contemporary forms of homophobia are rooted is therefore widely recognized in the literature on queer African sexualities (see, for example, Han and Mahoney 2018; Jijuuko and Tabengwa 2018; da Costa Santos and Waites 2019). In Ghana, the "against the order of nature" laws—also sometimes referred to as "sodomy laws"—that criminalized homosexuality during the colonial era can be traced back to Section 377 of the Indian Penal Code. This constituted the first "model" sodomy law of the British Empire and was instituted across many of Britain's African colonies (Human Rights Watch 2008).[10] These laws represented a key part of the regulatory mechanisms through which the "civilizing" impulses of the colonial project were legitimated and operationalized. While Ghana's laws were changed after independence, Section 104(1)(b) of Ghana's Criminal Offences Act essentially reproduces the colonial-era law. It prohibits "unnatural carnal knowledge," which is stipulated to include "sexual intercourse with a person in an unnatural manner or with an animal." "Unnatural manner" is not in itself defined, but it has been interpreted to include any form of penetrative sex that is not vaginal-penile, such as anal sex between men (Jeffers et al. 2010). Consensual unnatural carnal knowledge with a person aged sixteen years or over carries a charge of misdemeanor, with anyone found guilty facing a prison sentence of up to three years (Criminal Code of Ghana 1960).[11] Cases of unnatural carnal knowledge are difficult to prosecute due to the high standards of evidence required (Taylor Williamson et al. 2014), and there were few known arrests leading to prosecution in Ghana on the basis of the unnatural carnal knowledge law in the period 2013–2019 (Mendos 2019:328). Nonetheless, the existing law underpins a hostile juridico-political climate in which the arrest, imprisonment, extortion, blackmail, and intimidation of queer individuals— or those who are suspected of being queer—is commonplace. This climate would evidently become significantly more repressive in the event that the proposed anti-LGBTQ+ bill is passed.

In terms of the legacy of Britain's anti-homosexuality laws, Epprecht (2005) offers a compelling sociolegal genealogy of the Zimbabwean case, which excavates both the colonial roots of intolerance toward queer sexualities and shows how hegemonic constructs of masculinity (including expectations of heterosexuality) in white Rhodesian cowboy culture shaped the nationalist movement. This, in turn, laid the foundations for more contemporary expressions of homophobia, including President Mugabe's infamous 2011 claim that gays are "worse than pigs and dogs." Epprecht's genealogy differentiates temporally between the existence of heterosexist norms and attitudes— that is, the privileging of heterosexual relations, normative family models, and rigid constructs of masculinity and femininity—and the emergence of overtly homophobic ideas and values, as a means to historicize contemporary expressions of homophobia. A simplified version of this timeline in relation to recent developments in Ghana could be understood as comprising: a shift away from the post-independence context of entrenched heteronormativity whereby certain queer relations were nonetheless implicitly accepted (i.e., pre-1990s), toward a context in which homosexuality was increasingly politicized (i.e., from the late 1990s onward), culminating in increasingly forceful forms of politicized homophobia (i.e., post-2010) (see also Dankwa 2021).

Given the complexity of these shifts, Ryan Thoreson (2014:25) questions the value of the term "homophobia" in Africa, tout court, since it implies that such forces emerge from "fear rather than anger, hatred, bias, ignorance, jealousy, or other sources of antipathy toward queer persons." Thoreson (2014:26) further emphasises the plurality of homophobia, or "anti-queer animus," as he terms it, across different African countries, including contexts where it derives from "anxieties over pedophilia, recruitment, HIV/AIDS, denigration, pollution, and the fate of the nation," is "politically or religiously motivated," or forms part of "an apparatus privileging heterosexuality and reproduction while dismissing the validity of queer lives and relationships." I appreciate Thoreson's call for historical specificity in the study of heteronormativity and homophobia; that is part of my aim here. At a conceptual level, however, I am not convinced that homophobia's shortcomings necessitate a new framing, since it can be defined and contextualized in a way that addresses its diverse meanings and that enables precise analytical application. As set out in the first part of this chapter, this means understanding the relationship between the material and historical bases and drivers of heteronormativity (and particular sexual identities), the emergence of specific forms of politicized homophobia as a state strategy, the political economy of homophobic "moral panics," *and* how this shapes more cultural, everyday, and interpersonal manifestations of homophobia. In terms of types of homophobia, I would argue that it is a mix of all three examples outlined by Thoreson that underpins contemporary forms of politicized homophobia in Ghana; that is, politicized homophobia overlaps with anxieties over HIV, pedophilia, and national identity, is constituted by political and religious actors and discourses, and is rooted in a structural apparatus of heteronormativity that is (re)produced through state laws and practices, the organization of social reproduction, and norms regarding gender, marriage, family, and childbearing. This supports findings elsewhere in the literature that document how heteropatriarchal sex/gender regimes and articulations of homophobia have become increasingly encoded within the practices of postcolonial state-building across a number of African settings (Ndjio 2012; Rodriguez 2017; Currier 2018). Contextualizing country-specific dynamics of homophobia in Africa within these broader trends centralizes the ways in which statehood, citizenship, identity, and nationalism are configured in relation to normative and non-normative sexuality in the contemporary juncture. It also reveals why sexual and gender relations are a key site of political contestation and struggle (and a key vector of political values), and the impact of colonial antecedents and neocolonial power relations in the control and regulation of non-normative forms of sexuality and gender.

IN SEARCH OF "AFRICAN HOMOSEXUALITY"

Given the wide-ranging impacts of colonialism on gender and sexual relations in Africa, some queer (and queer-adjacent) scholarship has sought to document the precolonial existence of homosexual and other queer configurations of gender expression, eroticism, and intimacy. In this sense, it is homophobia, rather than homosexuality, that is the true (colonial and Christian) import (see Nyanzi 2015). As Thabo Msibi summarizes, "Same-sex desire can be traced before the arrival of Western people in Africa; homosexual behavior has always existed in Africa and continues to exist, though it was understood differently from the current construction of the West" (2011:72). This work builds on early pathbreaking collections by Stephen Murray and Will Roscoe (1998) and Ruth Morgan and Saskia Wieringa (2005), both of which highlighted the historical diversity of sexual and gender practices across the African continent.[12] Nii Ayen's contribution to the *Boy-Wives and Female Husbands* volume (Murray and Roscoe 1998) examined the complex cultural meanings attributed to MSM in West Africa. He suggests that Ghanaian society is characterized by a "code of silence" regarding sex that can be traced back to "Victorian, colonial and Christian ideas of what is 'prim and proper'" (Ayen 1998:125). Ayen's point about the effects of Christianity on Ghanaian gender and sexual norms is important and underscores not only how the colonial imposition of Christianity in Africa served to embed and legitimate imperialism (Bawa 2016:56), but the key role of sexuality within that process.[13]

Ayen's (1998) findings are further nuanced by Dankwa's (2021) research, which ties cultural norms of discretion and "indirection" in Ghana not to silence, per se, but to the linguistic practices of the Akan, Ghana's dominant ethnic group. In the Akan group of languages, metaphor, suggestion, and allusion are preferred over direct references, especially when it comes to "taboo" topics such as (queer) sexual acts and relations. Dankwa's (2021) analysis suggests that indirection should not be conflated with silence and that the "cultures of silence" narrative risks reproducing colonial tropes about African backwardness. It also reveals how cultural norms in Ghana that tacitly tolerated some queer intimacies and relations have undergone profound transformation, both during the colonial era and since independence, against a backdrop of political, economic, and social upheaval. This includes structural adjustment and ongoing processes of neoliberal economic reform, as well as the rise of African Pentecostalism, which reflects the wider revitalization of Christianity across the African continent (Klinken and Obadare 2018).[14]

According to Epprecht (2008:8), "The language by which same-sex relationships are described [in the academic literature] is often Eurocentric," primarily because homosexuality is used as a category for understanding sexual relations and difference in Africa. As a result, there has been a tendency for (some) academic and activist discourse to prioritize refuting the claim that homosexuality is "un-African," without sufficiently interrogating the meanings invested in homosexuality as a term and its (non-African) origins (Nyanzi 2015). No doubt, the homosexuality *is* African counternarrative may be politically expedient for activists seeking to address contemporary discourses of homophobia among political and religious elites, which center on the incommensurability of African culture and tradition with homosexual practices and desires. Similarly, its emphasis on the transformative impacts of colonialism on gender and sexual relations provides an important corrective to homonationalist framings that position "the West" as the global arbiter of LGBTI rights (Rao 2020). However, idealized accounts of precolonial queer relations, what Rao (2020) terms "homoromanticism," may not adequately address the social hierarchies, power relations, and political economic contexts in which these practices arose and, in so doing, may mobilize evidence of precolonial queer sexualities in rather anachronistic and instrumental ways. This dynamic evokes Macharia's (2009:157) critique of the ways in which "precolonial Africa becomes a foundation point of reference in adjudicating the status of contemporary attitudes and policies toward homosexuality." Put otherwise, in addition to acknowledging the role of colonialism and neocolonialism in producing the legal, political, and cultural contexts in which heteronormativity and homophobia are rooted and rearticulated, scholars must consider how and why contemporary discourses of homophobia have gained traction in some parts of the African continent.

Hoad (2007:xvi) proposes an alternative way of framing this debate, whereby homosexuality is understood as "one of the many imaginary contents, fantasies, or significations . . . that circulate in the production of African sovereignties and identities in their representation by Africans and others." This is a fruitful lens for exploring the politicization of homosexuality in the Ghanaian context, where homophobia has frequently been rationalized by Ghanaian politicians in terms of national sovereignty and by invoking essentialized ideas of "African" morality and culture (and where backlash is produced relationally, including through the interventions of Ghana's former colonial rulers, the British).[15] This is evidenced in President Mills's response to David Cameron's comments in 2011, when the United Kingdom was rebuked for "telling Ghana what to do" (Gray 2011). Although the politization of homosexuality has evolved since the gay conference and Cameron controversies of 2006 and 2011, concerns over sovereignty, morality, identity, and culture remain a unifying thread in presidential statements and other political discourse that opposes homosexuality and/or LGBTI rights.

The current president, Nana Akufo-Addo, led Ghana's main opposition party, the National Patriotic Party, to a narrow victory over the incumbent president, John Mahama, in 2016. In an apparent departure from the approach of his predecessor, Akufo-Addo made a number of early statements on the subject of gay rights.[16] In an interview with Al-Jazeera in November 2017, for example, Akufo-Addo told a reporter that the decriminalization of homosexuality was something that was "bound to happen" in Ghana and cited changes to the law in Britain as a case in point (GhanaWeb 2017). This provoked a fierce response from many MPs, including the Speaker of parliament, Aaron Mike Oquaye, who announced he would rather resign than oversee a debate on the decriminalization of homosexuality (GhanaWeb 2018a). Akufo-Addo subsequently sought to distance himself from his comments and to reassure religious and political groups of his commitment to "Ghanaian values." In 2018, Akufo-Addo's government released a statement explaining, "It will NOT be under his Presidency that same-sex marriage will be legalised in Ghana" (Shaban 2018). Since then, the president has come under further pressure regarding his position on homosexuality with the proposal of the anti-LGBTQ+ bill by members of the opposition party. Akufo-Addo's somewhat contradictory and shifting position on homosexuality, in the relatively short time-frame of his presidency, illustrates both how politicized homophobia in Ghana is evolving rather than static, and how it is constituted through a range of actors and forces, including those beyond the realm of formal politics.[17]

As this analysis suggests, any examination of the contemporary (and historical) roots of politicized homophobia in Ghana would be incomplete without acknowledging the key role played by religious leaders and institutions. Religious leaders were especially vocal during the "gay conference" controversy in 2006 and have continued to shape public debates over the so-called gay question. Reacting to the US Supreme Court ruling legalizing gay marriage in 2015, a host of Ghanaian religious leaders spoke out to denounce homosexuality: the head pastor from Emmanuel Assemblies of God counseled Ghanaians to "say no to same-sex marriage," calling homosexuality an "abomination" that goes against the "moral laws" of God (Daily Guide 2015a); the metropolitan archbishop of Accra, Palmer Buckle, argued that gay marriage should not be considered a human right and that "homosexual union means we don't want humanity to continue" (GhanaWeb 2015); and Reverend Isaac Owusu Brempah, from the influential Pentecostal church Glorious Word and Power Ministry, spoke out to urge the president to resist foreign pressure to decriminalize homosexuality (Daily Guide 2015b). Again, these interventions sought to depict homosexuality as a foreign import that goes against Ghanaian religious and cultural norms. They also implied that homosexuality, and relatedly gay marriage and LGBTI rights, endanger family, childbearing, and the future of the nation. The launch of a "national prayer crusade" against LGBTI rights by the Ghana Pentecostal and Charismatic Council in 2018, which included the establishment of "gay conversion camps" in major cities such as Accra and Kumasi (Daily Graphic 2018), indicates that the convergence and co-constitution of homophobia within political and religious spheres continues apace.

The national prayer crusade also illuminates how the landscape of queer sexual politics in Ghana has been reshaped by the rise of Pentecostal-Charismatic Christianity, both domestically and at the global level (Asante 2020). According to the 2021 census, Pentecostal-Charismatic Christians are the largest religious group in Ghana, representing 31.6 percent of the total population (GSS 2022).[18] Pentecostal-Charismatic churches typically espouse conservative and moralizing views on sexuality and gender, including opposition to premarital and extramarital sexual intercourse, as well as homosexuality. This discourse echoes efforts to control sexual behavior in Ghana made by early mission churches (Bochow 2008). As Asante (2020: 32) demonstrates, nineteenth-century colonial constructions of African sexuality as "pathological" and "degenerate" are similarly reproduced in contemporary Pentecostal-Charismatic discourses: in this context, they are displaced onto queer Africans. For Asante (2020), this highlights the ongoing coloniality of the Ghanaian Pentecostal-Charismatic Church (and the superficiality of their anti-imperialist posturing, as articulated through claims that homosexuality is un-African).

Pentecostal-Charismatic leaders propagate ideas about sexuality through church services and activities and through the Ghanaian media, as pastors participate widely in popular TV and radio discussions and write opinion pieces in mainstream newspapers (Bochow 2008; see also Dankwa 2021). This has contributed to the creation of what Astrid Bochow (2008: 402) calls a "sexualized public sphere." While there are various explanations for the popularity of Pentecostal-Charismatic Christianity in the contemporary West African context, its rapid growth during the 1980s has been linked to economic crisis (Deacon and Lynch 2013; Meyer 2007; Lindhardt 2015). The "prosperity gospel" thus appealed to particular sociodemographic groups because it offered both a spiritual and material response to economic and political turmoil (Deacon and Lynch 2013:109). At the same time, promises of economic prosperity have served to legitimate neoliberalism's "entrepreneurial subject" in moral and spiritual terms (Hackett 1999) and to rationalize a broader shift toward IMF-sponsored privatization and deregulation (Shipley 2009). This, according to Gregory Deacon and Gabrielle Lynch (2013:109), has undermined "class-based identification of and opposition to" the structural violence of the neoliberal era. These dynamics flesh out the account of homophobic moral panics set out earlier—in which religious leaders and discourse have played a key part—and further illuminates how these panics are connected to crisis, precarity, and rising inequality.

At a global level, right-wing US evangelical churches have documented links to prominent anti-gay clerics and churches in countries such as Uganda, Kenya, and Nigeria (Kaoma 2009). These links are economic as well as religious in character, as Kaoma (2009) explains: "Through their extensive communications networks in Africa, social welfare projects, Bible schools, and educational materials, U.S. religious conservatives . . . present themselves as the true representatives of U.S. evangelicalism, so helping to marginalize Africans' relationships with mainline Protestant churches." In the Ghanaian context, the ultraconservative Christian Right coalition World Congress of Families, which is based in the United States but has far-reaching global links, held a regional conference in Accra in 2019. The World Congress of Families seeks to promote "family values" around the world, including through opposition to abortion and equal marriage legislation. According to reports, the conference was attended by over five hundred delegates and included a session in which the organizers addressed the Ghanaian parliament "on the issues that weaken African traditional family values and how to confront them" (Catholic Secretariat of Nigeria 2019).[19]

US evangelicals are not the sole or even primary actor fueling homophobic moral panic in countries like Ghana and African clerics and other religious organizations have their own agency in colluding with parts of the US and global Christian Right (Rao 2020). Reporting undercover from the World Congress of Families conference in Ghana, Rita Nketiah (2019) noted: "Despite its US and Russian roots, this WCF summit felt distinctly African . . . the American presence was tiny, with notable exceptions" (namely the global president of WCF, Brian Brown). Nonetheless, human rights activists and journalists in Ghana have highlighted how the "family values" rhetoric of the WCF coalition, including its emphasis on expanded criminalization, is explicitly reproduced in the wording and aims of the anti-LGBTQ+ bill. They have further traced the WCF's links to the Ghanaian anti-LGBTI organization, the National Coalition for Proper Human Sexual Rights and Family Values (NCPHSRFV) (Rightify Ghana 2021), and highlighted the NCPHS-RFV's key local role in facilitating and promoting events like the 2019 summit (Nketiah 2019).

The NCPHSRFV was set up in 2013 by the prominent conservative and family values campaigner Moses Foh-Amoaning and has garnered support from a wide range of Christian, Catholic, and Muslim groups across the country. In addition to spearheading the anti-LGBTQ+ bill with a group of Ghanaian parliamentarians, the NCPHSRFV has previously been involved in organizing prayer and fasting events aimed at "fighting homosexuality legislation in Ghana," specifically gay marriage, and "praying the gay away" (GhanaWeb 2018b). Thus, while the precise contribution of the US Christian Right and events such as the WCF conference to the recent legislative proposals for expanded criminalization in Ghana is hard to quantify, it should be understood as one element within a heterogeneous coalition of transnational actors that are influencing and driving politicized homophobia.

This analysis has examined the critical role of the colonial and postcolonial state in Ghana in regulating and disciplining norms pertaining to homosexuality, including through legal prohibition. It has also explored some of the ways in which heteronormativity and homophobia are articulated through religious institutions and discourses in Ghana and pointed to the global and multiscalar character of these dynamics. This line of inquiry challenges reductive, Orientalist accounts that characterize "African homophobia" as a somehow timeless or transhistorical phenomenon. Rather, it foregrounds the political economic contexts that underpin homophobia, domestically and globally, and the constitution of politicized homophobia through interconnecting cultural, religious, political, and economic fields. I build on this discussion in the following chapter by looking at the impact of global HIV initiatives on the politics and organizational trajectory of Ghana's first formal LGBTI/HIV organization, the Centre for Popular Education and Human Rights Ghana (CEPEHRG).

CHAPTER 2

The NGO-ization of
Queer Activism in Ghana

Over the last five years, most of our funding is targeting HIV, condoms, lubricant, and everything. It looks like we are becoming more of an HIV organization than the LGBTI movement.
   —Evans-Love Quansah, executive director, CEPEHRG

In the development and global health literatures, scholars have identified the HIV epidemic as the key driver or "catalyst" for queer activism in the Global South (Roberts 1995) and in West Africa in particular (Nguyen 2005; Broqua 2015; Armisen 2016).[1] This chapter argues that this genealogy does not hold true in Ghana, where activists struggled for many years to develop and advance an organization primarily focused on LGBTI rights. As my case study of CEPEHRG, Ghana's first LGBTI/HIV organization, illustrates, these efforts were frustrated by a lack of resources, the politicization of homosexuality within the Ghanaian public sphere, and activists' growing entanglement in the global HIV response. This, in turn, has led to and accompanied processes of NGO-ization.

Adopting an HIV/sexual health focus was seen as strategically necessary by early activist groups like CEPEHRG in order to sustain themselves, in light of the funding and policy priorities of donors and the backlash and homophobia they experienced when pursuing more confrontational approaches to LGBTI rights. This homophobia was enacted through state institutions such as the government, the police, and the legal system, and became embodied in activists' everyday experiences of violence and discrimination. Despite this, many activists involved in the first wave of queer Ghanaian activism identify the narrow funding priorities and policy agendas of global development actors as the primary factor limiting their ability to build an "LGBTI movement." This sentiment is encapsulated in the comments from CEPEHRG's executive director Evans-Love Quansah that open this chapter.

Before looking at the politics of CEPEHRG in detail, I wish to spend a moment reflecting on the genealogy of these dynamics. To do so, I set out some of the broader shifts in development and global health policy that have shaped the terrain of queer politics in Ghana since the late 1990s and, I argue, transformed how queer activists organize around and frame their demands for LGBTI rights. I then focus on the specific case of CEPEHRG, delineating some of the key modes of organizing, political practices, and activities adopted by the group since its inception and documenting how the incorporation of HIV prevention and other sexual health rights work has (re)configured its political trajectory. This is evident in three main areas: aims and programmatic focus, understanding and approach to LGBTI rights, and organizational structures and practices. I trace these shifts to processes of NGO-ization, driven by neoliberal development paradigms at both the national and the global levels, which encourage professionalization, corporatization, and the adoption of (externally legible) organizational forms (Tsikata 2009).

Finally, the chapter explores the impact of politicized homophobia on formal queer activism and how groups organize (and *do not* organize) on LGBTI rights. These dynamics, I argue, necessitate an analytical approach that addresses not only how the political economy of development impacts formal civil society actors and LGBTI movement dynamics (for example, in terms of access to resources and processes of NGO-ization), but also how it works to (re)produce and reinforce structural inequalities, including class relations, heteronormativity, and homophobia.

HIV POLICY, KEY POPULATIONS, AND SEXUAL RIGHTS IN AFRICA

It is impossible to understand the genealogy of queer activism in Ghana without taking into account the growth of HIV initiatives targeting MSM across West, Central, East, and southern Africa over the last three decades. Across the African continent, national governmental responses to HIV have been steadily evolving (Makofane et al. 2013). This is characterized by improved understanding of the sociodemographic and geographic distribution of HIV, how this distribution is shaped by structural factors—poverty, gender inequality, homophobia, discrimination—as well as behavioral and clinical ones, and the development of appropriate and targeted interventions for those most at risk. While gaps in provision still remain, particularly in terms of preventative services for "key populations" (KPs)[2] and the availability of antiretroviral therapies and viral load testing (Ali et al. 2019), Ghana has led the way in what Akua Gyamerah (2021) terms a "paradigm shift" in continental HIV policy.[3] Amongst other things, this has entailed the recognition of transmission between men and the prioritization of MSM as part of the strategic response to the epidemic implemented by key national stakeholders, led by the Ghana AIDS Commission.

Moves toward targeted HIV interventions and the KP paradigm have dovetailed with the growing currency of "sexual minority rights" in the international domain.[4] The concept of sexual minority rights draws on decades of feminist, LGBTI, and antiracist activism and scholarship, and fits into a wider discourse of "sexual rights" (Akanji and Epprecht 2013). Sexual rights are not a discrete set of rights, per se, as they typically encompass human rights that have already been recognized in national laws and international and regional human rights agreements (World Health Organization 2017:3; Petchesky 2000). Moreover, there is no universally agreed definition of sexual rights, and the area has proved highly controversial within global policy and legal spheres. In development policy and practice, sexual rights are primarily framed as rights that are critical to the realization of sexual and reproductive health. According to the World Health Organization, for example, sexual rights include "the rights to the highest attainable standard of health (including sexual health) and social security; the right to marry and to found a family and enter into marriage with the free and full consent of the intending spouses, and to equality in and at the dissolution of marriage; the right to decide the number and spacing of one's children; the rights to information, as well as education" (World Health Organization 2017:3).

The Beijing Platform for Action, launched at the Fourth UN World Conference on Women in 1995, marked a key turning point in the evolution of sexual rights at an international level, with the concept becoming enshrined as a key constituent of women's human rights for the first time (Petchesky 2000). Since then, there has been a protracted and at times fractious struggle at the UN to broaden these rights to include sexual orientation and gender identity (SOGI) (Akanji and Epprecht 2013; Thoreson 2009). Key milestones in this process include the 2006 Declaration of Montreal, made at the first International Conference on LGBTI Rights; the development of the Yogyakarta Principles, also in 2006, which established a set of international legal principles relating to SOGI; and the publication of the UN General Assembly Declaration on Sexual Orientations and Gender Identity in 2008. Although non-binding, the UN declaration and Yogyakarta Principles reflect the changing status and growing legitimacy of sexual minority rights internationally (Thoreson 2009; Kollman and Waites 2009; Akanji and Epprecht 2013). In 2017, the African Commission on Human and Peoples' Rights adopted a landmark resolution on violence relating to SOGI, the first time the commission had explicitly pronounced on issues relating to LGBTI rights (Isaack 2017).

Global development agencies and donor governments were initially slow to take up the issue of sexual rights, especially those relating to SOGI. By the early 2010s, however, SOGI was becoming increasingly recognized as an important part of the global development agenda (Bergenfield and Miller 2014). The British, Danish, Norwegian, and Swedish development agencies— DfID, Danida, Norad, and Sida respectively—shifted their policy focus to include sexual and reproductive rights, and the Dutch government adopted an especially proactive role in prioritizing LGBTI rights.[5] Beyond Europe, the United States development agency USAID set out one of the most developed policy positions on sexual rights in 2014, including SOGI, and the Obama administration was outspoken on the need to promote and defend LGBTI rights around the world.[6] This included launching the Global Equality Fund in 2011, a "private-public initiative to support gay rights advocates around the world and to empower LGBTI persons." The Global Equality Fund operates through a coalition of NGOs, governments, companies, and foundations, and, according to its website, is "one of the largest sources of funding for the human rights of LGBTI persons" (2019).

In some senses, these shifts can be understood as a sea change in global development discourse, which has historically paid scant (rhetorical) attention to matters of sexuality. However, when evaluated at the level of development policy and programming, the scale and scope of change looks questionable, especially in terms of funding. Of the twelve largest development agencies in the Development Assistance Committee surveyed in 2014, for example, nearly all of them lacked any publicly available policy stating that aid would not be used by recipients to discriminate against LGBTI people or sexual minorities (Bergenfield and Miller 2014). The US government's declarations and initiatives, like those of other donor governments, have also not translated into significant amounts of aid money being channeled into LGBTI-specific rights work in the Global South. The Global Equality Fund, for example, spent just over $24 million in total—that is, across all regions—in small grants and technical and emergency assistance during the period 2011–2015. In the fiscal year 2015, it spent $10.9 million, with $2 million of this going to Africa. This is a drop in the ocean compared to the $284 million spent on foreign aid (excluding military assistance) in Ghana alone by the US government in fiscal year 2015, of which $77 million was spent on health and population assistance (USAID 2019). At an international level, in 2015–2016, $53.9 million of global funding was spent on LGBTI issues in "sub-Saharan Africa," with just $5.9 million (11 percent) of this going to West Africa, across all government and multilateral agencies, corporate funders, and public and private foundations around the world (Wallace et al. 2018:58). Again, this pales in comparison to the $10.2 million spent on HIV programming in Ghana by one single government agency, USAID, in the same year (USAID 2019).

The rather piecemeal character of efforts among the largest northern donor governments to address LGBTI rights is equally manifest within the United Kingdom's Foreign, Commonwealth and Development Office, formerly the Department for International Development (DFID). In 2017, DFID released the policy paper "DFID's Approach to LGBTI rights," a two-page document that committed the agency to promoting and protecting LGBTI rights, namely by "working with organisations in developing countries; building new relationships; and utilising evidence to support change." This was not a new strategy, per se, since this was already integrated into the department's existing approach: as the paper states, "This work will be taken forward through our existing 'inclusive development' work." Indeed, this approach had de facto characterized DFID's work for some time. DFID's Uganda Operational Plan, published in 2014, similarly identifies LGBTI rights as a key issue of concern, primarily in relation to the Ugandan government's proposed anti-homosexuality legislation.[7] Yet it commits DFID to only two actions: "lobbying the government to oppose any efforts to introduce new anti-homosexuality legislation" and "designing a DFID-funded, FCO- [Foreign and Commonwealth Office] managed project on LGBTI rights engaging the Police, Human Rights Commission and NGOs" (DFID 2014:19). Again, this stands in stark contrast to the amount of donor resources dedicated to sexual health. The United States and the United Kingdom are the first and third largest donor countries to global health respectively (with Germany in second place), through both bilateral and multilateral arrangements, such as the Global Fund to Fight AIDS, Tuberculosis and Malaria. To add some further context to this, $2,427 million of the United Kingdom's health Official

Development Assistance (ODA) in 2021—the latest year for which full data is available—was spent on health, approximately 15 percent of the United Kingdom's total ODA in 2021 (donortracker 2023).

As the above figures suggest, the United States has continued to be a major financial player in the global response to the HIV epidemic, as part of the President's Emergency Plan for AIDS Relief (PEPFAR), especially in Africa. In Ghana, much of the funding for HIV work among MSM has come through USAID and, more recently, the Global Fund. Two USAID-funded projects were especially significant in establishing MSM-targeted activities in Ghana: the Academy for Educational Development's Strengthening HIV/AIDS Response Partnerships program (frequently referred to as "SHARP"), which began in 2004, and the Strengthening HIV/AIDS Response Partnership with Evidenced Based Results, or "SHARPER," program, a follow-up project to SHARP implemented in 2010 (Gyamerah 2017). USAID's decision to support bilateral targeted HIV prevention activities among MSM in Ghana was informed, in part, by the publication of the "Ghana Men's Study" (Robertson 2009:5; Attipoe 2004), which documented the extent of HIV prevalence among MSM in the country. This controversial report not only provided empirical evidence of the existence of MSM in Ghana, their elevated rates of HIV, and the presence of a concentrated epidemic among this group, but directly challenged the Ghanaian government to address the issue strategically in its HIV policy. While the inclusion of transmission between MSM was not formalized in national policy in Ghana until 2011, some seven years later (Gyamerah 2017), the publication of the 2004 Attipoe study, the shifting focus of HIV prevention efforts among funders like USAID, and mounting evidence of MSM's disproportionate vulnerability to HIV infection, effectively transformed the landscape of queer politics in Ghana, especially for small activist organizations like CEPEHRG.[8]

Speaking to some of the most long-standing activists involved in HIV and LGBTI rights work, it is clear that the rollout of programs such as SHARP and SHARPER and the longer-term repositioning of Ghana as a "model" African country in HIV policy has been highly contested. This is, in part, because the biomedical rationalities that underpin these types of HIV response have marked queer men as a key target and site of intervention, as a public health risk and "at risk" group, and as a discrete, nominalized, and increasingly visibilized section of the population. While the Ghanaian case evidently has its own specificities, the country is, in many ways, a microcosm of broader struggles around HIV, the KP paradigm, and LGBTI rights in Africa. As

described in the previous chapter, one key part of this picture is the politicization of homosexuality within the Ghanaian public sphere, which has, since
the 2010s, transmuted into intensified forms of politicized homophobia. This
constitutes a state strategy tied to contestations over nationalism, identity,
and sovereignty in the context of postcoloniality, as well as global trajectories
of political economic transformation and crisis. At the same time, the politicization of homosexuality has been relational to, and bound up with, the
growth of NGO and other community-based activism on LGBTI and sexual
health rights.

THE ORGANIZATIONAL TERRAIN OF SEXUAL RIGHTS ACTIVISM

From the late 1990s onwards, a small handful of organizations began working on HIV prevention and sexual and reproductive health advocacy among
MSM in Ghana, both in the capital Accra and in other major cities. Some of
these organizations included an explicit focus on LGBTI rights. In addition
to CEPEHRG, the organization Maritime Life Precious Foundation was established in Takoradi in the early 2000s. Maritime Life Precious Foundation
provides health education and poverty reduction strategies to communities,
including MSM, on the western coast of Ghana and, like CEPEHRG, received
funding through the USAID-SHARP program from 2004 to 2009. More recently, Solace Brothers Foundation was launched in Accra in 2012, with the
aim to "advance human rights and sexual reproductive health rights for LGB-
TI persons in Ghana," and, in 2015, Samuel Adjei, a former peer educator
and long-standing advocate for MSM health rights, set up the NGO Priorities
on Rights and Sexual Health (PORSH). Although PORSH is not explicitly
focused on LGBTI rights, it aims to "attain equal rights and privileges in life
for vulnerable sectors of society," which includes MSM.[9] In addition to these
groups, the NGO Human Rights Advocacy Centre (HRAC) is another important organizational actor in the field of human and sexual rights.[10] Established in 2008 by the Ghanaian lawyer and former minister for gender,
children, and social protection, Nana Oye Lithur, HRAC seeks to promote
and protect human rights across a number of key areas, including gender-
based violence, sexual and reproductive health, and what it terms "minority
rights," which includes rights for LGBTI people. Historically, HRAC has been
the only medium-sized national NGO in Ghana to include this type of "minority rights" in its programming and advocacy work. Accordingly, it has of-

ten worked in collaboration with smaller groups such as CEPEHRG. Notable examples of collaboration include the organization of annual Pride events, programs to mark International Day against Homophobia and Transphobia, and the rollout of "values clarification" workshops with healthcare service providers and police personnel on discrimination toward LGBTI individuals, and specifically MSM.[11]

HIV PREVENTION AND SEXUAL HEALTH RIGHTS: TRANSFORMING FIRST-WAVE ACTIVISM

As their organizational names and objectives indicate, groups like CEPEH-RG, Maritime Life Precious Foundation, PORSH, and Solace Brothers Foundation have prioritized sexual health rights, which, in practice, largely entails HIV prevention and advocacy work for MSM. Yet the history of CEPEHRG, Ghana's first LGBTI/HIV organization, reveals that the HIV epidemic was not the primary catalyst or politicizing force in its work. Prior to setting up CEPEHRG, Evans-Love Quansah undertook a training program in popular education and human rights organized by the British Council in Accra. It was this training, he told me, combined with his passion for improving the lives of queer people in Ghana, that led to the establishment of the group. According to Evans, the road to establishing CEPEHRG as a formal organization was long and difficult, and he encountered resistance from key institutional and civil society actors all along the way. One example of this was the Registrar General Office's refusal to recognize Evans's group as an LGBTI organization in the early 2000s. Evans tried various different names, including the "Gay and Lesbian Association of Ghana" and "Friends of Dorothy," both of which were refused by the office. Ultimately, he opted for CEPEHRG, which contains no explicit mention of LGBTI rights.

In our interview, Evans made it clear that CEPEHRG's intention in the early days of organizing was to focus on issues relating to sexual orientation. Over time, however, the organization began to increasingly incorporate HIV and sexual and reproductive health work into its remit. According to Evans, this shift was related to the aid funding climate at the time, which forced the organization to specialize in the area of MSM health. The USAID-funded SHARP program, which began in 2004, was particularly significant in this regard. Facing a difficult political climate and resistance to the Most at Risk Populations approach (later renamed the KP approach) among key national stakeholders, USAID's SHARP team sought to recruit implementing partners to work with the target populations—female sex workers and men who have sex with men—on the ground (Eveslage 2015). In the Greater Accra region, this group was CEPEHRG.

Writing about West Africa, Mariama Armisen (2016:10) suggests that HIV interventions on MSM created the first formal queer organizing spaces in the region. These spaces gave peer educators the opportunity to evolve, over time, into activists. While it is certainly true that a number of Ghanaian activists started off in HIV prevention work, in CEPEHRG's case, it was the other way round, with a combination of factors prompting CEPEHRG to change its focus. This included a lack of funding opportunities for LGBTI rights initiatives; a shift in policy and programmatic interest among donor governments, development agencies, and later the Ghanaian government toward HIV and the KP approach; and experiences of violent backlash when activists engaged in more public and visible advocacy efforts focused on LGBTI rights. While the pressure to "specialize," as Evans termed it, was accompanied by growing recognition on CEPEHRG's part of the impact of HIV and other STIs on queer men in Accra, the group's core political priorities at the time lay elsewhere.

In terms of its LGBTI rights work, over the years CEPEHRG has provided human rights and security training to staff, peer educators, and other queer individuals, released statements advocating LGBTI rights and the protection of queer individuals during moments of homophobic moral panic, such as the David Cameron controversy in 2011, run community theater events for LGBTI individuals, and produced advocacy materials relating to LGBTI rights. In addition to these activities, CEPEHRG has formed alliances with other LGBTI/MSM organizations and allies, such as Maritime Life Precious Foundation and HRAC.

CEPEHRG's community theater workshops aim to explore human rights abuses relating to gender and sexuality. Although community theater was originally conceived as a means to reach out to LGBTI populations, CEPEHRG subsequently adapted it to engage with and educate the wider public on issues relating to HIV prevention. This strategy has been helpful in facilitating access to communities where more visible attempts to meet with groups of MSM are considered too dangerous. Moving into more general sexual and reproductive health programming has also allowed CEPEHRG to broaden its programmatic focus and to access additional funding opportunities. This discreet and pragmatic approach to LGBTI rights advocacy substantiates, in some respects, Epprecht's (2012) argument that African LGBTI activists are using sexual rights models in innovative and adaptive ways, notably by embedding LGBTI rights within heterosexual public health initiatives in order to bring about subtle and incremental change. Certainly, for Ghanaian groups like CEPEHRG, adopting a flexible and responsive approach has enabled it to carry out various forms of rights-based and health-oriented activities over the years, to establish new funding sources and transnational partnerships, and to open up new fields of intervention. This, to borrow Currier and McKay's (2017) terminology, would be characterized as a "hybrid strategy," which combines both "public health" and "social justice" approaches to activism.

While it is important to recognize innovation and adaptability in the use of sexual health rights paradigms (and how development agendas are transformed and repurposed by activists on the ground), there are a number of issues that complicate this line of analysis in the case of CEPEHRG. First, as staff members repeatedly pointed out, CEPEHRG's decision to move its focus from LGBTI rights toward health-oriented activities was very much related to—perceived and actual—development funding opportunities and a lack of donor interest in LGBTI rights work. In essence, this constitutes less a hybridization of LGBTI rights and HIV than a move away from LGBTI rights to HIV prevention. This transformation is evidenced in the decreased frequency of popular education, consciousness-raising, and other specifically LGBTI rights-focused activities since 2000 and the organization's downscaling of attempts to incorporate "lesbian" and other queer women into its organizing. During my fieldwork in 2013–2014, for example, I observed only two community events that used these approaches to reach out to LGBTI individuals. Over time, this shift has resulted in a growing sense of anger and confusion among some community activists and peer educators about the core priorities of the organization and the extent to which LGBTI issues are being marginalized. As I show in the following chapter, these shifts, articulated through a broader process of NGO-ization, have engendered growing disconnection and division between CEPEHRG and the communities the organization seeks to represent.

No doubt, working on HIV prevention among MSM remains a highly politicized activity in and of itself in Ghana, particularly given the elevated levels of societal stigma directed toward both queer people and people living with HIV. On the one hand, then, HIV research and program activities conducted as part of the KP paradigm have contributed to the *politicization* of homosexuality within the Ghanaian state. On the other, the move toward formalized, NGO-ized modes of HIV service delivery has entailed a set of *depoliticizing* effects on first-wave activist groups like CEPEHRG. This is evident in relation to their organizational objectives (e.g., prioritizing project and target-based objectives tied to HIV prevention, as opposed to more radical or structural forms of political change relating to LGBTI rights) and organizational structures and practices (e.g., premised on corporatization and the "professionalization" of staff, which in turn increases reliance on development funding).[12]

THE NGO-IZATION OF RESISTANCE

CEPEHRG's trajectory of formalization parallels trends across other parts of West and East Africa, where many LGBTI groups have increasingly adopted the governance and financial models of non-profit and non-governmental organizations in the Global North (Theron et al. 2016; Rodriguez 2019; see also Roy 2016). While these models vary according to the legal norms in different country settings, they typically share four characteristics: corporate governance and leadership structures, corporate finance and human resource management practices, ongoing monitoring and evaluation of program activities, and a grassroots base for accountability, with responsibility for shaping long-term policies and strategies (Theron et al. 2016). As Theron et al. (2016) note, these processes frequently result in the prioritization of donor agendas over the needs of grassroots queer communities. This ties in with longstanding feminist critiques of NGO-ization in the Global South, including in Ghana, which highlight how this works to depoliticize, deradicalize, and co-opt social movements (Tsikata 2009; Castro and Hallewell 2001; Roy 2016).

Sabine Lang (2013:62) defines NGO-ization as "a shift from rather loosely organized, horizontally dispersed and broadly mobilizing social movements to more professionalized, vertically structured NGOs." It is rooted in shifting state-market relations under neoliberalism, notably the rolling back of the state in the provision of welfare and other key social services (and the rolling out of civil society as a means to fill the gap) (Choudry and Kapoor 2013). In this new policy context, NGOs are understood as key vehicles "for fostering democracy and the creation of new markets" (Keshavjee 2014:7). State-civil society partnerships have therefore been promoted by global development actors such as the World Bank and the United Nations since the 1990s as part of the "good governance" agenda (Sharma 2008). While processes of NGO-ization are multiplex and geographically differentiated, they are reflective of the ways in which neoliberal logics have increasingly shaped relations between social movements, NGOs, state institutions, and other governance bodies.

One obvious example of this in Ghana is the dominance of the sexual health agenda in development and how this has reshaped the political and programmatic focus of groups like CEPEHRG. In addition, the adoption of formal organizational structures has resulted in a more top-down, technocratic, and managerialist approach and prioritization of upward accountability mechanisms, that is, a concern for reporting and responding to funders, as opposed to their grassroots base. This shows how the "politics of recipiency," to borrow Nora Kenworthy's (2017:25) phrase, is operating in Ghana, but here it is transforming the relationship between HIV/LGBTI NGOs and their bases (i.e., in addition to broader state-citizen relations). S.M. Rodriguez (2019:107) observes similar dynamics in Uganda, where the bureaucracy of transnational LGBTI organizations, advocacy, and funding, they argue, "divests from alternative forms of organizing, and instead reinvests in small networks of power that center around the most powerful institutions and governments in the world." While Rodriguez (2019) documents growing factionalism and competition between queer activist groups as a result of NGO-ization, in Ghana, it has resulted primarily in internal discord and division. Indeed, for CEPEHRG, dynamics of corporate restructuring and managerialism have begun to seriously trouble their relationship with grassroots queer communities, including their own network of peer educators. As Musah, a former peer educator who established his own sexual health rights group, explained:

> At the end of the day, even though they target LGBTs, peer educators are classified as third-class citizens. LGBTs, gays especially, are third-class citizens.

To illustrate the "third class" treatment of LGBTI individuals, Musah recounted a story from a peer educator training event:

> There was a time when we had a program outside Accra and we were in the hotel. About four or five of us went to the swimming pool. Doing our own thing, swimming, being ourselves and that stuff. Within an hour, we heard, "Are you fools? What are you doing? Look at the way you dress and now at the

hotel they are also going to tag us as if we are gay. If you want people to tag you, OK. But then don't let people tag us because we are not one."[13]

This experience of verbal abuse—in an environment that was intended to bring together queer men to learn about sexual health rights—was very upsetting for Musah and was, he told me, one of the incidents that prompted him to set up his own group. In this way, dynamics of NGO-ization should be understood to both encompass and engender deep-rooted tensions between community and organizational strands of queer organizing and within the alliance of HIV, sexual health, and LGBTI rights. This includes tensions over the disciplinary and at times gender-normative attitudes of NGO staff, perceived class differences and therefore a sense of economic inequality between NGO workers and peer educators and other community activists, and frustration over the health-dominated nature of these organizations' agendas.

Musah is not alone in expressing anger toward Ghana's formal LGBTI/HIV organizations, with peer educators and other community activists repeatedly emphasizing their disillusionment with NGO-led interventions on HIV and LGBTI rights, especially peer education. I examine this strand of Ghanaian LGBTI/HIV organizations' work in detail in the following chapter. However, if there is perhaps one phrase that sums up these feelings of anger and disillusionment, it is the line, "And they sit there in their air-conditioned offices," which I heard frequently during interviews, informal conversations, and participant observations over the course of my research. Like Musah's comments, this reflects a sense of class anger among activists, a sense that NGO jobs, even in a small organizations like CEPEHRG, are well remunerated and therefore more middle-class positions, and that the work (and perhaps the lived experience) of NGO staff is easier than that of working-class activists. In a context of entrenched inequality, high unemployment and underemployment rates, and pervasive poverty, this reveals how the NGO-ization of resistance interacts with and reproduces power relations relating to class and sexuality. As Gabriel, another peer educator, commented ruefully, "Some of them [NGO workers], they think they are the class type. Class. Class. Class." These feelings of anger are further compounded by the hierarchical and managerialist attitudes displayed by some NGO workers toward peer educators.[14]

Evans-Love Quansah's testimony indicates, however, that formal LGBTI rights activism in NGOs like CEPEHRG is far from easy work. Moreover, many of the experiences of homophobia described by working-class community activists are echoed in the accounts of CEPEHRG staff. This suggests that the political economy of development—the way in which neoliberal funding mechanisms and donor agendas create top-down models of accountability, instill performance-centric management and financial practices, and disconnect NGOs from grassroots queer communities—serves to individualize struggle and reinforce class divides. While I might distinguish between smaller NGOs like CEPEHRG that are carrying out advocacy work on MSM and LGBTI rights and do employ queer people as staff, and larger national NGOs and government actors, these distinctions were not frequently made by peer educators and other community activists in their criticisms. This finding reveals how powerfully queer working-class men's experiences of subordination and oppression inform their perspective and speaks to what Jon Binnie (2014:241) terms "the transnational dimensions of classed sexualities". In other words, it is these material conditions, class relations, and inequalities that provide the primary lens through which community activists interpret the political economy of HIV response, irrespective perhaps of some of the more contradictory dynamics on the ground.

UNEASY ALLIANCES: CEPEHRG AND STATE-CIVIL SOCIETY RELATIONSHIPS

As part of their transformation into a formal HIV organization, CEPEHRG has also been drawn into a broader set of state-civil society partnerships centered around national HIV response. According to staff members, the alliance between LGBTI/HIV organizations like CEPEHRG and national policy stakeholders like the Ghana AIDS Commission has been a profoundly uneasy one, in part due to their divergent political agendas and incentives. As Kweku Aborah, a staff member at CEPEHRG, noted, reflecting on the motivations of key national policy stakeholders such as Ghana AIDS Commission:

> They still have their judgmental comments and attitudes that they pass about these people behind their back. But then because it is a business that they are doing and because money comes out of it, they are pretending.

In Kweku's view, national policy actors are primarily motivated by the anticipated financial rewards attached to MSM-targeted HIV work—namely donor money—rather than any "passion for LGBTI rights," as he puts it. The idea that "it is a business" locates HIV prevention for MSM within the political economy of development aid, whereby funding streams such as PEPFAR/ USAID are big business for Africa's expanding civil society sector, as well as serving key strategic and geopolitical functions for both recipient countries and donor governments in the Global North (Gary 2007; see also Chan 2015). In Kenworthy's (2017:25) work on Lesotho, she refers to this as a "politics of recipiency," whereby HIV funding streams have effectively transformed governments' relationship with development actors, shifting state accountability away from citizens toward donors. This politics goes some way to explain the seemingly contradictory policy position adopted by the Ghanaian government, in which it has sought to promote the sexual rights of MSM through targeted HIV interventions and government institutions like the Ghana AIDS Commission, while continuing to criminalize homosexual relations and promote increasingly vehement anti-gay sentiment. Evans reflected on this contradiction:

> We've had challenges with homophobic people working on HIV prevention for MSM just because the money is there. We've had challenges where people push money that is supposed to go to LGBTI groups to groups that are not LGBTI-specific, because they don't want to actually empower an LGBTI movement. We've had challenges where they tell you they will work with you for five years saying, "We're building their capacity." And then they will finish with you after five years and say, "They have no capacity."

Here Evans highlights how donor-funded HIV prevention work has compelled activists to work alongside, rather than in opposition to, hostile—and, at times, openly homophobic—government and civil society actors. It has also prioritized predominantly health rights (as opposed to LGBTI rights), and specifically queer men's health rights (rather than those of lesbians, other queer women, transgender, and otherwise gender non-normative individuals). These trends reinforce and reproduce the marginalization of queer women's needs and voices within global development discourse (Gosine 2006), as well as the assumed "invisibility" of queer intimacies and relations between women in contexts like Ghana (Dankwa 2021). Evans's comments about capacity-building also highlight the limitations of development funding that is contingent on the adoption of vertically organized corporate structures, professionalized practices, and other technocratic reforms and how this impacts the long-term sustainability of organizations that do not, for whatever reason, comply with these imperatives.[15]

At a practical level, the mixed motives and agendas of different stakeholders makes CEPEHRG's programmatic and policy work particularly fraught, since it is effectively required to shapeshift as an organization depending on context. Whereas in some circumstances CEPEHRG emphasizes its work with KPs—in documents or materials intended for donors such as USAID and the Global Fund, for example, or in its work with the Ghanaian government on HIV—in other contexts it clearly identifies its work in terms of LGBTI rights—for example, in relation to its involvement with AMSHeR (African Men for Sexual Health and Rights), a regional African coalition for grassroots MSM and LGBTI organizations. These pragmatic acts of self-representation allow CEPEHRG to navigate multiple (and competing) spheres of intervention and interest: global and national public health initiatives, local and regional activist networks, conservative institutional and national civil society networks, grassroots queer communities. Yet they also reveal how profoundly CEPEHRG's activism is mediated by institutional homophobia (as in the case of its work with the Ghanaian government, where it typically downplays its LGBTI rights work) and political economy (as in its relationship with donor agencies, where it tailors and refashions its organizational remit according to the dominant development agendas and funding streams du jour).[16]

Evidently, it would be simplistic to reduce CEPEHRG's development as an organization solely to questions of funding, as significant as this might be to staff members and peer educators. Rather, CEPEHRG's organizational trajectory has been shaped by an array of factors, which includes the shifting continental and global policy context around HIV and sexual rights, processes of NGO-ization linked to neoliberal development paradigms, and the domestic politicization of homosexuality. I look at these dynamics in more detail in the following section, with a particular focus on the backlash, threats, and violence the group experienced following a public campaign intended to promote LGBTI rights in Ghana in the early days of its organizing.

BETWEEN ACCOMMODATION AND RESISTANCE

The forms of political activity adopted by CEPEHRG have historically steered a careful line between accommodation and resistance, caution and confrontation. By organizing community-level sexual health outreach programs for MSM, engaging in popular education and awareness-raising activities among MSM populations, and incorporating LGBTI rights issues into more general sexual and reproductive health rights initiatives, CEPEHRG has largely avoided direct confrontation with homophobic political and institutional actors and power structures. CEPEHRG's collaborative work with other NGOs such as HRAC, which includes initiatives such as human rights sensitization workshops for LGBTI individuals, and the West African AIDS Foundation, which includes running a sexual health drop-in clinic, has also tended towards non-confrontational approaches. Rather, these collaborations have been used as a platform to provide services or programs to MSM and LGBTI individuals or to support behind-the-scenes advocacy work on human rights in HIV and sexual and reproductive health policy.[17]

In the decade between 2010 and 2020, the few occasions where CEPEHRG spoke out publicly on issues relating to LGBTI rights were responses to homophobia in the public sphere, as in 2011, for example, when they released a statement on President Mills's condemnation of LGBTI rights and professed commitment to the criminalization of homosexuality in Ghana. In this instance, CEPEHRG organized its response through the Coalition against Homophobia in Ghana (CAHG), which describes itself as "a group of organizations and individuals that aims to counter ongoing attacks against homosexuals in Ghana." As part of this initiative, CAHG came out to "vehemently denounce these types of sensationalist, unfounded, and bigoted attacks against LGBTI Ghanaians" (Valenza 2011). Given the extremely volatile political climate at the time, which saw a series of homophobic attacks on queer individuals and groups in Accra, this was a bold and potentially dangerous action by CEPEHRG and their allies. Notably, however, CAHG did not explicitly detail the members of the coalition in their public statement, an omission that reveals how, even in this more direct political intervention, they continued to prioritize safety and pseudonymity.

In lieu of more explicit, targeted actions that aim to confront or change state laws and policies, CEPEHRG have sought to build the human rights knowledge and consciousness of queer individuals and communities in Accra carefully, discreetly, and "from the ground up," as one staff member put it. This cautious approach is reflected in the organization's mission statement, which, like its name, is worded to avoid any specific mention of LGBTI rights. Moreover, its website includes a long list of areas of specialism: "Human Rights, Advocacy, HIV-AIDS, Gender Sensitization, Research, Training,

Performances, Children's Rights, Popular Education, Women's Rights, Civil Activism, Counselling, Democracy and Good Governance, Minority Rights, Peer Education, Documentation, and Information Dissemination." Buried toward the end of this list, "minority rights" is not further defined.

At the time of my research, the organization's offices are similarly discreet: enclosed within a walled compound and guarded by a watchman, only a small, faded sign bearing the acronym CEPEHRG identified the space. Talking to CEPEHRG staff, it is clear that much of this caution resulted from the harassment, violence, and abuse staff members have experienced as a result of their activism. CEPEHRG staff reported repeated incidents of intimidation, threats, attempts at blackmail and extortion, and verbal and physical abuse in response to their activities. These incidents have caused a great deal of trauma and distress and, for some staff members, have left them in a state of fear and paranoia.

It would be valid, in some senses, to conceptualize these oscillations between visibility and invisibility in the language of movement strategy, that is, as part of CEPEHRG's toolkit of organizational approaches or tactics. However, I think this more technical social movement terminology obscures the ways in which activism and resistance are embodied in and shaped by more microlevel and everyday experiences of oppression and violence. Put otherwise, lived experience sediments into CEPEHRG's organizational practices and priorities, as part of what I would term the corporeality of activism. These experiences are not necessarily verbalized or translated into concrete strategies or policy documents; rather, they form the basis of an implicitly agreed-upon set of practices that help a small group of individuals navigate an extremely challenging political landscape, in which instances of moral panic over homosexuality have become increasingly commonplace.

ACTIVISTS, MORAL PANICS, AND POLITICIZED HOMOPHOBIA

There is no doubt that the gay conference controversy of 2006 marked an important watershed in both public discourse surrounding homosexuality in Ghana and the approaches to LGBTI rights advocacy adopted by activist groups like CEPEHRG. It cast unprecedented media spotlight on the activist known as "Prince Macdonald"[18]—the spokesperson who raised the topic on JoyFm radio—and triggered a sustained anti-gay backlash that is clearly etched in the memories of many activists I met in Ghana. For CEPEHRG staff, the backlash they experienced in 2006 was both frightening and formative; staff members were followed, encountered gangs waiting for them in public spaces, were subjected to protests from religious groups calling for homophobic violence, had their cars vandalized with the tag "Burn it up," and received death threats. As a result, CEPEHRG was forced to move offices from Accra's central commercial district of Osu to a quieter area outside of the city center. It also began adopting a much more discreet and nonconfrontational approach to LGBTI rights activism.

This offers an important insight into the way in which the political economy of development interacts with politicized homophobia in Ghana to systematically limit the activities of queer activists. These limitations are constituted through activists' extensive encounters with homophobia and violence, their experiences of backlash when they adopt more direct forms of political action (as in the example of the radio appearance), their limited access to resources, and their inability to obtain significant donor support to maintain and fortify LGBTI rights work. CEPEHRG's unsuccessful attempt to register the NGO with any reference to LGBTI rights is another case in point, indexing the symbolic impossibilities of queerness in the face of heteronormativity and state power, here in terms of homophobic institutional actors like the Registrar General.

At a more personal level, these experiences have wide-ranging implications for activists' mental health and well-being, since conducting LGBTI rights work and being publicly out in Ghana takes a heavy emotional toll. As Evans commented, "It is seriously psychologically challenging to be living an openly gay life here." For some CEPEHRG staff, these difficulties have led them to modify aspects of their lifestyle to conform more closely to norms of masculinity and to avoid detection by friends and family. I examine the mental health impacts of homophobia in Chapter 4 of this book.

UNDERSTANDING LGBTI RIGHTS: A "HOLISTIC" APPROACH

One notable feature of first-wave queer political organizing has been its historic reluctance to challenge the existing legal framework surrounding homosexuality in Ghana. In lieu of a comprehensive set of LGBTI rights—which might include, for example, decriminalization or anti-discrimination laws—organizations like CEPEHRG, PORSH, and HRAC advocate what they refer to as a "holistic" approach to rights that aims to work within the existing parameters of the law. To an outside observer, this partial conceptualization of rights may appear confusing. Yet, much like CEPEHRG's development as an LGBTI/HIV organization, it is very much rooted in the lived experience of activists, as this has been shaped both by politicized homophobia and their incorporation into development initiatives on HIV and sexual rights.

Since 2011, CEPEHRG has remained largely reticent on the question of decriminalizing homosexuality, a position that has similarly adopted by PORSH and HRAC. Broadly speaking, these organizations' approach to rights has emphasized that LGBTI Ghanaians should enjoy the same rights as other Ghanaian citizens, as enshrined within the Ghanaian constitution. For CEPEHRG, this is articulated as a means of recognizing the rights of LGBTI people without giving them what they term "special rights." As Evans explained:

> At a point we realized that it might not even be the best to be talking about the rights of LGBTI persons. Because human rights are enshrined as part of our constitution for everyone. So then advocating for LGBTI rights means sometimes it's interpreted as looking for special rights for LGBTI people.

Evans's comments about interpretation refer to public perceptions of queer activists and the risk of backlash. The idea that "human rights are enshrined as part of our constitution" suggests that legal reforms are not essential to realizing LGBTI rights and, on its website, CEPEHRG explains the universality of human rights *without* specific mention of sexuality, sexual orientation, or gender identity:

> Everyone can claim human rights, despite: a different sex; a different skin colour; speaking a different language; thinking different things; believing in another religion; owning more or less—being born in another social group; coming from another country; and any other differences that may occur between us. (CEPEHRG 2019)

This represents an important strand in first-wave organizations' understandings of LGBTI rights: the "holistic" approach. This is a specific conceptualization of holistic, not to mean the full gamut of LGBTI rights, but rather the "whole" set of rights as provided for Ghanaian citizens under current law. One of my interviewees, a former executive director of HRAC, sought to further distinguish between "LGBTI rights" and, what he termed "the human rights of LGBTI people." Again this distinction may sound confusing or even sophistic, but for HRAC it is an important one since it allows activists to pragmatically negotiate rights, to contest rights violations, and to assert citizenship under the current auspices of the law.

According to Samuel Adjei, founder of PORSH, this holistic approach reflects the realities of the Ghanaian context and, above all, the entrenched forms of homophobia that act as a barrier to queer liberation:

> LGBTI rights in isolation to me is difficult to understand in our context because we are not there yet. We are not in a place where we can segregate rights. We are nowhere near LGBTI rights in the next five years. Where we are is to take human rights as holistic and then dovetail them under human rights.

In this way, PORSH argue for the same approach proposed by CEPEHRG and HRAC, in which LGBTI rights are folded into—"dovetailed under"—a broader framework of human rights that does not explicitly focus on SOGI.

For these organizations, advocacy around LGBTI rights in Ghana does not comprise or necessitate calls for the decriminalization of homosexuality or claiming other formal LGBTI rights, such as equal marriage. As Jacob, another staff member at CEPEHRG, argued:

> More often than not it [LGBTI rights] is misconstrued as though we are saying we should legalize same-sex sexual activity or same-sex marriage. But that is not it. If we are talking about rights, the fundamental rights of every human being should be respected, irrespective of his sexual orientation, creed, age, religion, what have you. So you do not expel somebody from school simply because he's LGBT. A landlord or a landlady does not evict someone from his home because he's LGBT. If somebody comes with a boil in the anal area, you do not start standing on the moral high ground, preaching. You are a medical professional and you have to do your job.

Jacob identified three key areas where LGBTI individuals should be able to exercise rights: education, health, housing. Protection from discrimination on the grounds of sexual orientation or gender identity in these areas is, in his view, a key defining element of LGBTI rights. However, these protections are not understood as an explicit claim to sexual citizenship—in terms of citizenship based on recognition of formal equality before the law, or on certain protected characteristics such as sexual orientation—but as an assertion of the basic rights that are enjoyed by any Ghanaian. This follows a similar logic to the "holistic" argument set out above, with Jacob emphasizing that the decriminalization of homosexuality should not be considered a priority for queer Ghanaian activists.

While not all the organizational activists I interviewed espoused fixed views on the question of decriminalization, very few identified changing the unnatural carnal knowledge law as a current political priority. Instead, the primary concern for groups like CEPEHRG, PORSH, and HRAC was typically articulated as securing better protection in terms of accessing services and living without violence. As Evans explained:

> We need a law which protects people and strengthens how people build the capacity of these minority groups. That's what we need in place to make sure you can walk in for services and know that nobody can attack you on the way. Because nobody has the right to attack anybody. Nobody will insult you because nobody has the right to insult any other person because he's a minority.

Evans argued that any legal reforms should seek to protect minority groups from violence, which, in turn, will enable them to access services. Significantly, however, Evans did not link access to services or the right to live free from violence to decriminalization, but referred to a "modification" of the existing law that would ensure protection and improve capacity-building among LGBTI individuals. When I asked him directly about his position on the unnatural carnal knowledge clause, he clarified:

> I will not say the Unnatural Carnal Knowledge law should be changed. But then there should be a law that helps provide equality, equal access to services and other things.

Kobby Mensah, an experienced HIV outreach worker and program manager at Maritime Life Precious Foundation in Takoradi, highlighted how the existing legal framework is used to target and intimidate queer men, even in cases that are unlikely to lead to conviction:

> I've seen a case where people were put in police cell for three months, ninety-two days, you know, because even though the police didn't have the evidence, they rushed the case to court, committed the case to court and kept on saying

that "look, since the case is in court there's nothing really we can do." Because the case has been started and courts processes over here is very, very, very slow.

According to Kobby, the men were targeted because of their involvement in grassroots queer organizing. Evidently, it was a very intentional move on the part of the police:

> I remember the police investigator telling me that he has heard that these people are organizing gay community members and he will make sure he breaks that community organizing. That's why he's doing that. He's not doing that for the sake of the law.

Even for Kobby, however, these experiences do not necessarily mean that LGBTI/HIV organizations should be calling for changes to the unnatural carnal knowledge law. Rather, he again sees it as a case of enacting and using the existing laws of the constitution, namely around the freedom to self-expression and the right to privacy; as he put it, it is about "fully operationalizing the rights regimes that go by the tenets of the constitution."

There is little doubt that the politicization of homosexuality in Ghana over the past two decades has had a profound effect on organizations' willingness to pursue confrontational forms of queer organizing. However, formal LGBTI/HIV organizations' hesitance around—and in some instances outright rejection of—calls for decriminalization in Ghana also reflect some of the contradictions that inhere to some of the broader contradictions that inhere in public health approaches to addressing sexual injustice, which have both embedded human rights as the primary framework for articulating political demands and delimited their parameters. As Makofane et al. (2013) note, while transmission between MSM has been increasingly recognized in HIV national strategic plans (NSPs) in Africa, many of these plans fail to acknowledge the key role of criminalization and other human rights violations for MSM in driving the epidemic. While Ghana's 2010 NSP does recognize that the criminalization of homosexual activities presents "obstacles to access to prevention, treatment, care and support" (Ghana AIDS Commission 2010:69), the idea of conferring rights to gay men or decriminalizing homosexuality in Ghana has continued to be met with fierce resistance among key state and non-state stakeholders in HIV response (Gyamerah 2017:132).

Insofar as the tensions that arise from strategies of selective inclusion—access to rights in some areas and continued discrimination and exclusion in others—are evident to prominent LGBTI/HIV organizations, they also seem to have been accepted, to some degree, as part of the internal logic of sexual health rights work, where connections between the legal and institutional architecture of homophobia and oppression and the ways in which homophobia is enacted and reproduced in everyday sociocultural contexts are not consistently drawn. This logic is articulated in multiple ways, as in the idea of a "holistic" approach to LGBTI rights, and is powerfully reinforced by activists' personal experiences of backlash, violence, and homophobia. It is similarly manifest in CEPEHRG's attempts to prioritize the right to live free from violence, for example, while at the same time distancing itself from claims to what it sees as explicitly LGBTI rights, including decriminalization. This supports Susie Jolly's (2007) observation that "negative" articulations of sexual rights in development—that is, those that focus on public health, danger, and risk, as opposed to more "affirmative" rights such as protection from discrimination or equality—may work to disempower activists in the Global South, namely by bolstering conservative ideologies concerning sexuality and reinforcing homophobic stereotypes. In this instance, this dynamic is operating at a much more micro level, shaping how formal LGBTI organizations conceptualize these issues and how they claim (and do not claim) rights.

AN UNCERTAIN FUTURE

The case of CEPEHRG, Ghana's first and most prominent LGBTI rights group, troubles genealogies of queer African activism that take the HIV epidemic as the sole or primary point of departure. The group's trajectory illustrates instead how sexual health interventions and global HIV response have impacted, transformed, and ultimately constrained the field of queer politics and organizing—notably by pushing organizations to formalize and specialize in HIV—as well as activists' struggles to advance LGBTI rights in the face of politicized homophobia. Of great concern among activists at the time of my research was a potential shift in the legal framework governing LGBTI rights, namely the expanded criminalization of homosexuality, as seen in other African states such as Uganda and Nigeria.[19] Sadly, this possibility has since materialized, in the form of the anti-LGBTQ+ bill. This bill builds on previous efforts by the leader of the National Coalition for Proper Human Sexual Rights and Family Values (NCPHSRFV), Moses Foh-Amoaning, to fortify the law's existing prohibitions on homosexuality. In 2018, the NCPHS-RFV sought to introduce a parliamentary bill entitled A Comprehensive Solution Based Legislative Framework for Dealing with the Lesbianism, Gay, Bisexual, and Transgender (LGBT) Phenomenon. This included a proposal to categorize homosexuals into two classes, "penitent" and "irredeemable," and to offer prayer, counselling, and healthcare treatments to those who fall into the first category. Those homosexuals understood to be beyond help, that is, irredeemable, should, according to the NCPHSRFV, be prosecuted using the full extent of the law (McCabe 2018). While the 2018 bill was not ultimately debated within parliament, it marked an important shift in tactics from the NCPHSRFV, which included the adoption of more "secular" and "pseudoscientific" language and a focus on legislative reform (Martínez et al. 2021:95).[20]

Against this background, there is little doubt that formal LGBTI/HIV organizations in Ghana face a challenging and unpredictable future. Part of this relates to scale, since the activities of CEPEHRG and other groups are reliant on extremely small networks of people and, in some instances, single individuals. This has significant implications for sustainability, not least because of the emotional toll taken by the work and the high degree of risk it entails. A second key part of this relates to the divisive and contradictory impacts of HIV interventions on existing queer political formations, as well as their broader role in intensifying forms of politicized homophobia. These dynamics have engendered a growing divide between formal, NGO-ized spaces of queer organizing and more grassroots, community-based ones, as I explore in the following chapter.

HIV Prevention, Peer Education, and Queer Labor in the Global Development Industry

As for MSM interventions, it's not theory. It's not just theory, you sit there in your office and write reports. No, it's pure practical work. You have to talk to a person and, you will know, it's very difficult.

—Marcus Lamptey, former peer educator, CEPEHRG

Against a backdrop of politicized homophobia, the shift toward sexual health programming among first-wave LGBTI organizations in Ghana has offered clear financial and security-related advantages. Yet it has also brought about processes of specialization (i.e., in HIV prevention), formalization, and NGO-ization. For CEPEHRG, this has meant changing its strategic aims and the types of issues it prioritizes, as well as how it organizes as a group. Specifically, CEPEHRG's sexual health work requires the organization to mobilize networks of queer men across parts of southern Ghana to carry out front-line HIV prevention activities on a voluntary and unpaid basis, referred to as "peer educators." This model has been adopted by other long-standing HIV organizations working with KPs and is foundational to community-level HIV prevention efforts in the country.

Peer education interventions have been implemented extensively across the Global South since the 1990s (Medley et al. 2009). Peer educators are typically engaged by NGOs on a voluntary basis to carry out HIV prevention activities and other sexual health outreach work among populations disproportionately affected by HIV, including MSM and female sex workers. The World Health Organization (2012:21) defines peer education as a "community empowerment-based intervention" for which "the benefits are high, there are no harms and the required resources are relatively low." This chapter explores whether these initiatives are indeed "empowering" and "harmless" for the queer working-class men who work as peer educators in Ghana's capital city, Accra. It also considers how these interventions impact on the wider terrain of queer political organizing in this context. Theoretically, I do so by reading peer education through the lens of social reproduction, that is, as part of the "life-making" activities that are systematically devalued (and frequently invisibilized) within the global capitalist economy (Bhattacharya 2017).

In Ghana, peer education models were roundly criticized by current and former peer educators for relying on the voluntarism, that is, unpaid labor, of working-class men. Anger over inadequate compensation and recognition for the work was compounded by poor accountability mechanisms and a perceived lack of representation within Ghana's formal LGBTI/HIV organizations. Peer educators thus contrasted Ghana's growing international reputation as a model African country for its HIV policy with the harsh realities of life as a queer person in Accra, which include wide-ranging experiences of homophobia, violence, discrimination in housing and employment, homelessness, poverty, and social exclusion. These dynamics have left peer educators feeling frustrated and exploited. Building on the case study of CEPEHRG set out in Chapter 2, the following analysis reveals how queer men's work in peer education fuels and reinforces the divide between formal and informal strands of HIV/LGBTI and other forms of queer activism—that is, between the more middle-class spheres of civil society and the working-class queer networks of Accra—places a disproportionate burden of responsibility for tackling the HIV epidemic on queer working-class men, and increases peer educators' risk of homophobic violence and abuse.

The chapter begins with Adam's story, a former peer educator who has grown increasingly disillusioned with sexual health rights advocacy and NGO-led approaches to queer struggle. Against this background, the chapter explores the implications of queer men's entanglement in development interventions on HIV and their work as peer educators, drawing connections to gender equality initiatives and the women's empowerment paradigm. In so doing, it locates peer education within the activities and lineages of social provisioning, caring, and other affective labor that have been historically uncounted and undervalued in the global economy and sets out how this relates to contemporary shifts in global development discourse, namely the emergence of a neoliberal empowerment paradigm. To do this, the chapter examines three key issues raised by activists in relation to peer education programs in Ghana: voluntarism, compensation, and accountability and representation.

"IF THE THING IS TOO HEAVY FOR ME TO CARRY, I WILL CARRY·IT BY FORCE"

It is early Sunday evening and I have arranged to visit Adam Amoah, a former peer educator, at his place in Mamprobi, a suburb to the west of Accra, out past the Korle Lagoon. We have met a handful of times before, in some of the queer-friendly bars in Jamestown and as part of a group discussion with peer educators a few weeks earlier. Wearing shorts, a cropped pink T-shirt, and a pair of orange *chalewɔte*,[1] Adam apologises for not being dressed. He tells me that he spent the day resting and watching DVDs and lost track of time. His room is narrow and there is no space for chairs, so the three of us, Adam, my research assistant Edward, and I, sit down on his single mattress.

Adam is twenty-eight. He is one of those people who looks both much older and much younger than his years. Friendly and softly spoken, he listens carefully as we go over the details of the interview. After we finish, he turns to talk to my research assistant in Ga, a playful grin spreading across his face as he recounts an anecdote about one of his neighbors. Despite his upbeat manner, I sense that Adam has a lot on his mind; the warmth of his smile belies something more melancholic and his attention flickers on and off unpredictably, like the little electric lamp he uses to light up the yard.

Adam was born in Accra, in a busy compound house he shared with his mother and sisters. Adam's father is Akan, but he left when Adam was young and Adam was raised speaking Ga, the native language of his mother. Adam was very close to his family as a child, his sisters in particular, and there were always people around him in the house: aunties, uncles, cousins, and other relatives. Despite his "feminine mannerisms," Adam told us he was popular in school, joking and clowning around to entertain his classmates. He was also a talented singer and active in his local church. He sang solos in services and performed in the church choir all through his childhood and teenage years.

Adam became sexually active when he was thirteen, with another boy from his neighborhood. He continued to have queer sexual encounters as a teenager, but strove to keep his sexuality a secret from his family. At the age of twenty-one, Adam became seriously involved with an older married man. "He was my first love. I came to love him even more than my siblings." They were together for around a year, before his boyfriend got sick. Adam tried to look after him as best he could. "I took him to the hospital and paid for his care and all that. The love was there." Despite efforts to treat him, after a short period of illness his boyfriend passed away. For Adam, the exact cause of his death was never clear. The loss of his partner hit Adam hard and he decided to stop dating for a while.

It was during this time, when Adam was around twenty-three, that he discovered he had a sexually transmitted infection, something he assumed was anal warts. Adam was reluctant to go to the health clinic. Stories of queer men facing stigma and homophobia from health workers were commonplace among his friends, and he was fearful of people finding out. Adam tried to treat the condition himself but, unsure of the diagnosis, the medicines he took just seemed to make it worse. Bleeding heavily and in a lot of pain, Adam was forced to seek medical attention. The doctors advised him he would need an operation. The procedure they carried out, he says, did not resolve the problem, and his health continued to deteriorate. In and out of hospital and struggling to pay the mounting medical fees, Adam began losing weight. With the weight loss came the gossip. "You know the way our friends are, if you become slim a little, there will be so many perceptions." Once part of a wide social network, Adam found that his friends and acquaintances began to withdraw from him. "So I became like a prodigal son who has been sent away from home. I had to go back to where I came from because I didn't have anyone to help me."

It was at this point that Adam returned to his family home to seek support. Again, however, he found that his dramatic weight loss was affecting his relationships, this time with close family members. So too were rumors of his sexual relations with men. "They sacked me.[2] They told me I should go to my husbands who are having sex with me to look after me." Rejected by his family and feeling increasingly isolated, Adam turned to an older queer woman known within the community as "friendly to *sassoi*." By this time, doctors had confirmed something Adam had feared for a while: he was HIV-positive. Adam paused as he told us this, glancing over to look at my research assistant and me. Edward smiled and nodded gently and, without saying anything else, Adam continued with his story. He told us that he stayed with his friend, his auntie as he called her, for a few months. According to Adam, she gave him the emotional support he needed to seek treatment and get back on his feet: "She didn't have money to help me, but there are people whose words make you happy."

Adam had since moved to a single room in a different part of town. He had been able to reestablish relations with two of his siblings, but he still felt a profound sense of loss and isolation. "My beauty is lost. I have lost my stature. Every day I am becoming smaller." He was also unable to access regularly the medicine he needed to manage his HIV and struggled to stay optimistic. Lonely and frightened, his thoughts turned often to suicide and death. "I am always in my room. I don't go near anyone to be asked any questions."

At the end of our interview, I asked Adam about his fears and concerns for the future. He said he worries about how he will die and the stigma, gossip, and loneliness he imagines lie ahead. "The way in which *sasso* dies is that you become slim, you become disoriented, and people say things they shouldn't say about you." He continued, "People are not dying a physical death. People are dying in a way like, people need people."

Two things that gave Adam the motivation and courage to carry on are his queer friends and support networks and, importantly, his activism. "The pains I am passing through, I don't wish my friend or brother to go through that. So I have been helping people." Adam said he would like like to do more to support other queer men like him, but he lacked the financial resources to do so: "I don't have money. But I am praying that one day money will fall like manna." There was a spirituality to Adam's words, as he went on to explain the personal strength he thinks queer activists need to keep going. "Because me, *iye noko ye imli* [I have something inside me]. *Iye spirit ko ye imli ni tamɔ* [I have some spirit inside me]. Even if the thing is too heavy for me to carry, I will carry it by force."

Adam's moving account of life as a young queer person in Accra highlights some of the intimate links between community activists' experiences of violence and hardship and their commitment to helping others. Adam's comment that *sassoi* die in a particular way—"you become slim, you become disoriented, and people say things they shouldn't say about you"—evokes the idea of HIV enacting a form of "social death," to borrow Judith Butler's (2004:29) phrase, that prefigures the physical one. It is this rejection by friends and family, both actual and anticipated, that Adam finds the most difficult part of living with HIV and, as a result, a key motivator in his activism. Adam's political will—the "spirit inside him"—is bound but not foreclosed by these dynamics. This almost contradictory relation—the tension between structure and agency—is encapsulated in Adam's poignant avowal, "If the thing is too heavy for me to carry, I will carry it by force."

The lived experience of men like Adam is not simply about inadequate healthcare, HIV, or stigma. Rather, it reflects the complex ways in which macrolevel political economic forces sediment down to the individual and micro level, becoming embodied in both personal stories of suffering and everyday practices of resistance. It is these forces—institutional homophobia, criminalization, discrimination, and economic inequality—that not only produce the conditions in which HIV is much more likely to affect queer working-class men in Ghana, but structure a whole range of other violations and indignities: stigmatization, homelessness, unemployment, poverty, social exclusion, loneliness, isolation. In order to fully comprehend sexual health interventions premised on peer education, we need to attend to this broader context of oppression and injustice and to consider how this impacts, in a systematic way, on men like Adam, who represent both the intended benefi-ciaries *and* the frontline providers of HIV prevention services.

Adam worked as a peer educator for CEPEHRG for nearly three years. When I first met him in 2014, however, he had recently given up peer edu-cation work to focus on what he called his community activism. Like many activists I spoke to, Adam was deeply critical of the forms of voluntarism that sustain peer education work in Ghana, whereby local development organiza-tions use volunteers to carry out health promotion, testing and counselling, and other preventative HIV services. While community activists identified wide-ranging issues with the operationalization of peer education programs in Ghana, their overarching concern related to the terms and conditions of the work, in particular, the extent to which it was unpaid, unrecognized, and often dangerous for the men involved. These experiences, I argue, hold important insights into the political economy of the global HIV response and how queer men's caring labor is deployed within this context.

THE WORK OF A PEER EDUCATOR

In Ghana, peer educators are employed on a voluntary basis to carry out HIV prevention and other sexual rights outreach work among MSM. According to the Ghana AIDS Commission's standard operating procedures (2014:63), MSM peer educators are responsible for "day-to-day community outreach activities; providing information, education, and services to their peers in project sites; compiling weekly narrative reports; and mobilizing KP (Key Populations) for prevention, care, and / or treatment educational programs." As this short description suggests, peer educators play a central role in HIV prevention and sexual health outreach work among KPs and the standard operating procedures go on to specify an extensive range of duties that peer educators are expected to carry out. This comprises over twenty separate ac-tivities, many of which are linked to specific metrics, for example:

The provision of one-on-one and small group sessions on HIV prevention

Condom and lubricant demonstration and sales

Conducting basic risk assessments and providing information on referrals to HIV testing and counseling (HTC), STIs, anti-retroviral therapy (ART), and other services

Provision of information on sexual and gender-based violence, reducing drug and alcohol use, and building self-esteem

Participation in refresher training

Referral of KPs for STI services

Accompanying KPs to facilities providing STI services

Referral of KPs for testing and counselling services

Accompanying KPs to facilities providing HTC services

Referral of all KPs that test HIV-positive to an ART clinic

Promotion of KP HIV-positive support groups

Organizing one-on-one monitoring sessions

Organizing small-group discussions on behavior change communication (BCC)

Organizing condom and lubricant use demonstrations and sales each month

Distribution and usage of BCC materials. (Ghana AIDS Commission 2014:63)

The level of detail in this job description, for what is essentially a volunteer role, is striking. Moreover, as Gyamerah (2017:241) documents, when these job responsibilities are cross-referenced with the minimum package of services set out in the key populations standard operating procedures, peer educators are given "the most responsibilities in carrying out the minimum package of services in MSM HIV/AIDS efforts," across all service providers and implementing partners.

As part of their employment, peer educators receive a stipend, locally known as an allowance. At the time of my research, this was approximately 240 cedis per month (equivalent to around forty British pounds). The allowance is intended to cover travel expenses, as well as any other costs arising from the work. While the Ghana AIDS Commission's more recent standard operating procedures state that "PEs [peer educators] can be engaged on a stipend *or as fully paid staff members* depending on the financial capacity of the implementing partner" (2018:17, italics mine), I encountered no fully paid peer educator staff members during my research. In terms of monitoring and evaluation, peer educators are expected to fulfill certain weekly and/or monthly quotas, which are set and agreed upon by implementing partners, in light of the overall targets and objectives specified by the funders for each intervention. These quotas pertain to indicators such as number of new KPs reached, number of condoms distributed, number of peers accompanied to an STI clinic for testing, number of KPs referred for STI testing, and number of KPs referred for HIV testing and counseling (Ghana AIDS Commission 2014). The peer educator's performance is then monitored and evaluated against these metrics through various mechanisms, namely field observations, monthly review meetings, and the submission of weekly reports.

There is a lack of good-quality data on the effectiveness of peer education interventions in Africa (Beyrer, Baral, et al. 2012; Shangani et al. 2017). The evidence base is especially limited when it comes to assessing the impact of individual and group-level interventions on reducing HIV transmission (Beyrer, Baral, et al. 2012) and on increasing testing in low- and middle-income countries such as Ghana (Shangani et al. 2017) (as opposed to other metrics such as increased knowledge of HIV and other STIs, where peer education interventions have proved more successful). Gyamerah (2017) documents issues in data quality pertaining to the reach and impact of MSM interventions in Ghana. In this instance, however, I am less interested in the health-related impacts of MSM peer education programs, as important as they are from an epidemiological perspective, than in the extent to which peer education is realizing its wider objectives of "community empowerment."

HIV PREVENTION AND "COMMUNITY EMPOWERMENT"

Empowerment is a nebulous, "elastic" concept in development discourse (Cornwall 2016:342). While the concept has a long history in feminist activism and social movement organizing, it has become increasingly disconnected from its more radical roots as it has been incorporated into mainstream development policy and practice (Batliwala 2007; Cornwall 2016). According to Andrea Cornwall (2016:342), empowerment is one of the most slippery of development's buzzwords, not least because it has been taken up and rearticulated by a heterogeneous "coalition of corporations, global non-governmental organizations, banks, philanthrocapitalists and development donors." Within the field of HIV prevention, the embrace of community empowerment approaches has a similarly complex background. As Vinh-Kim Nguyen (2010:25) explains, the approach was initially informed by the experiences of northern HIV/AIDS activists in the 1980s, particularly in North America, where involving the gay community and people living with HIV was understood as central to achieving public health outcomes. In this context, patient empowerment and community-led health interventions were developed by activists seeking to push back against the biomedical establishment at the time, which was seen as both homophobic and technocratic. These initiatives also reflected a broader social environment in which the "medicalization" of health and disease was viewed suspiciously (see also Chan 2015). At the same time, the Anglo-American model emphasized the importance of "coming out" as living with HIV, a set of practices premised on collecting (and quantifying) HIV testimonials that Nguyen (2013) broadly terms "confessional technologies."

As these technologies were globalized, HIV testimonials came to represent a key way of measuring the success of African governments' HIV response and, therefore, of adjudicating whether or not to maintain aid funding. Nguyen's analysis illustrates how empowerment approaches to health promotion operate in Africa, where the translation and application of HIV policies and practices developed in the Global North is profoundly mediated by neoliberal rationalities, including in aid funding. Moreover, the technologies they rely on are often ill-equipped to deal with complex and varying political, economic, and social realities on the ground, including, in Ghana, the growth of politicized homophobia. As Colleen O'Manique (2004:9) observes in the Ugandan context, this means that "the pandemic is still overwhelmingly viewed first and foremost through a biomedical lens, and secondly through a narrow public health lens that focuses on individual sexual behaviour."

THE POPULARITY OF PEER EDUCATION APPROACHES

While health promotion discourse since the 1980s has increasingly adopted the language of "community empowerment," the underlying theoretical rationale for peer education has not always been consistently or clearly defined (Turner and Shepherd 1999). Typically, peer education has been associated with ideas of credibility, empowerment, reinforcement, and role modeling (Turner and Shepherd 1999), as well as cost-effectiveness. It has also been grounded in behavioral change theory (UNAIDS 1999). More recently, the empowerment dimension of peer education has taken on even greater prominence, whereby peer education approaches are specifically rationalized as models of community empowerment (see UNAIDS 1999; Population Council 2000; Campbell and Mzaidume 2001; World Health Organization 2012). The World Health Organization's claims that peer education is highly beneficial, harm-free, and cost-effective (2012:21) is perhaps understandable if assessment is based exclusively on health-related metrics among target groups (although, as noted above, the evidence base on this is at best patchy). However, given the extremely challenging climates in which many MSM and female sex worker peer educators are working across the Global South (and parts of the Global North), which includes criminalization, stigmatization, politicization, and elevated risk of violence, this seems like a problematically partial assessment. It also highlights the extent to which the impacts of peer education approaches on peer educators themselves, that is, as a discrete group of individuals (and *workers*), have not been routinely or systematically evaluated, especially in the African context.[3]

What does emerge clearly from the health policy literature—and documents like the WHO guidelines—is that, in addition to empowerment, a key part of the popularity of peer education approaches is their perceived cost-effectiveness, primarily because they do not use fully qualified or trained health-care personnel (UNAIDS 1999; World Health Organization 2012; Hutton et al. 2003; Pinkerton et al. 1998). In this sense, they are consistent with the broader neoliberal imperatives of downscaled public service provision and upscaled reliance on civil society actors. A number of these underlying assumptions and principles can be discerned in Ghanaian HIV policy and practice. The Ghana AIDS Commission National Strategic Plan (2016: 94–95) identifies the protection of both the "social and economic" and "human" rights of KPs as part of its core strategies, which are to be achieved through a range of activities, including support for community advocacy (for example, by providing "technical assistance and material support" to "CSOs [Civil Society Organisations] and PLHIV [People Living with HIV] associations' advocacy on promoting and protecting the rights of KPs"), stigma and discrimination reduction programs, and identifying and establishing links with other "pro-poor economic and empowerment assistance" schemes. While the protection and promotion of rights for KPs is a laudable commitment, in reality, this has been hampered by the ongoing prohibition of homosexual relations between men in Ghana and entrenched forms of institutional homophobia, including among key national stakeholders. These barriers and constraints also mean that, in practice, it is the biomedical and individual-level aspects of behavior change—partner reduction, condom usage—that continue to provide the cornerstone of HIV prevention interventions among MSM in the country. This pattern is reflected in HIV prevention and AIDS-care related research and interventions across the Global North and South more generally (Kaufman et al. 2014).

The community empowerment-related principles and objectives of peer education are thus located within a shift toward "empowerment" approaches in global development discourse, which in turn constitutes an evolving set of neoliberal governance practices. As Lynn Haney (2008:25) explains, "the socioeconomic projects of neoliberalism are frequently promoted as empowerment projects. . . . It is precisely this promise of empowerment that makes neoliberal forms of governance so effective and resonant". When viewed in this light, the connections between the issues raised by activists involved in peer education work in Ghana and the normative underpinnings and short-comings of women's empowerment programs, discussed in detail in the next section, are clear. Of central concern here is the extent to which mobilizing queer men's caring labor through forms of voluntarism is unfair and exploitative—given the lack of employment opportunities, limited access to labor markets, discrimination, and homophobia they experience—and how this links to the broader (re)privatization of care under neoliberalism.[4]

Within the academic literature, an emerging corpus of studies has examined the politics of MSM interventions and their implications for local queer communities and identities (Boyce 2007; khanna 2009, 2011; Boellstorff 2011; see also Gosine 2013). This scholarship provides useful insights into the opportunities and constraints of MSM as a sexual/epidemiological category and rights-bearer in development policy (and what this means across different spatial and temporal contexts). It also shows how MSM interventions have manifold and often unintended effects, including politicizing, visibilizing, and reifying marginalized communities that already face discrimination and stigmatization. However, this literature has not typically conceptualized peer education as a form of queer labor, nor has it considered the links between neoliberal development processes, relations of social reproduction, and the provision of preventative HIV services for MSM more generally.[5] In the following section, I examine these dynamics through the lens of social reproduction and in relation to two key phenomena: the emergence of a neoliberal empowerment paradigm in global development discourse and shifts in the organization of social reproduction across the Global South.

THEORIZING QUEER MEN'S CARING LABOR IN DEVELOPMENT

Since the 1970s, a wealth of feminist scholarship has sought to render visible the role and value of social reproductive labor within the global capitalist economy (e.g. Vogel [1983] 2013; Laslett and Brenner 1989; Katz 2001; Bakker and Gill 2003; Federici 2004; Bezanson and Luxton 2006; Bakker 2007; Fraser 2016; Bhattacharya 2017; Ferguson 2019). At its most basic level, social reproduction is defined as "the maintenance of life on a daily basis and intergenerationally" (Laslett and Brenner 1989:382–383), with women understood to bear a greater burden of social reproductive labor than men. Black feminists, alongside other scholars working in the Black radical tradition, have documented the extent to which social reproductive labor is racialized and territorialized in character (i.e., as well as gendered), and how relations of social reproduction have been violently disciplined and instantiated, through slavery, colonialism, and shifting regimes of capitalist accumulation (Davis 1981; Hill Collins 1998; Hartman 2006; Bhattacharyya 2018).

In order to clarify how we might conceptualize peer education in this context, Catherine Hoskyns and Shirin Rai's (2007) expanded definition of social reproduction is useful. In this account, social reproduction entails "biological reproduction; unpaid production in the home (both goods and services); social provisioning (by which we mean voluntary work directed at meeting needs in the community); the reproduction of culture and ideology; and the provision of sexual, emotional and affective services" (Hoskyns and Rai 2007:300). According to this definition, the unpaid, voluntary labor that undergirds HIV prevention programs can be understood in terms of its social reproductive function, since it encompasses the provisioning of care and affective services at the community level. This work is neither fully privatized since it does not take place exclusively within the family or through kinship networks, nor fully socialized, since it is supported by civil society actors who do not cover all the costs, particularly in terms of labor.

The emergence of a "care crisis" in the Global North is another significant area of debate within the feminist social reproduction literature (Bakker and Gill 2003; Hoskyns and Rai 2007; Fraser 2016). Broadly speaking, this argument holds that, as provisioning in child, health, and social care has been rolled back, the costs of—and responsibility for—social reproduction have been increasingly transferred from the state back onto individuals and households, through a process of "reprivatization" (Bakker 2007; Bakker and Gill

2003). The care crisis is rooted in the deep, structural contradictions of maintaining and reproducing life under contemporary modes of financialized capitalism and represents one facet of a multidimensional "crisis of social reproduction" (Fraser 2016). While the salience of the "reprivatisation" thesis has been questioned in countries like Mexico (Kunz 2010), across much of Africa, social reproduction has been characterized by similar patterns of commodification and crisis, albeit in this context through structural adjustment and other forms of neoliberal restructuring in the context of postcoloniality (Ossome 2021).

In Ghana, the social welfarist policies of the post-independence era gave way to deep public spending cuts and sweeping market-oriented reforms during the 1980s, followed by continued market liberalization in the 1990s (Konadu-Agyemang 2000). This entailed the systematic introduction of user fees in health care: a so-called cash-and-carry system that resulted in widespread health inequalities and poor health outcomes for large swathes of the population (Abukari et al. 2015). It is in this context that women's unpaid "private" care work (and the household more broadly) has been understood as a crucial "shock absorber" for the effects of structural adjustment programs (Elson 1992), providing, as O'Manique (2004:8) puts it, "the 'cost-effective' underpinning of market freedom." This landscape of limited state provisioning, inadequate health infrastructure, widening inequality, and ongoing crises of social reproduction—which have been exacerbated by the HIV epidemic—is also the context in which queer men have found themselves increasingly co-opted into multiscalar HIV response.

The fact that many low- and middle-income countries have been in receipt of substantial foreign development aid targeting areas like basic healthcare might appear, at first glance, to complicate this trajectory of privatization and commodification. Since the early 2000s, the growing currency of the "good governance" agenda has seen, amongst other things, the prioritization of poverty reduction efforts alongside economic development, typically orchestrated through national-level "poverty reduction strategy papers" (PRSPs).[6] However, while this aid represents significant direct investment, it has been distributed and operationalized according to the structural and policy prescriptions of the Washington Consensus, namely the downsizing of the state and the public sector and, in so doing, the upscaling of civil society, which has been positioned to fill the void, albeit with a fraction of the financial capacity (Ruckert 2010).[7]

Feminist scholars of development have long documented how the types of poverty reduction and gender equality interventions that proliferated within development policy in the 1990s impacted on social reproduction. One key policy change from the structural adjustment era was an increased role for civil society and turn toward the language of women's "empowerment" (Molyneux 2006:429). In practice, however, conditional cash transfer programs and microfinance initiatives served to advance the commodification of women's labor power, intensify the unequal division of labor, and reinforce patriarchal gender norms (Chant 2008; Molyneux 2006; Parpart et al. 2002). Significantly, these programs frequently relied on women's voluntarism, resulting in what Sylvia Chant (2008:187) calls the "feminization of responsibility and/or obligation". By sourcing women's productive labor on a voluntary basis (and not addressing their disproportionate responsibility for social reproductive labor), economic empowerment programs have paradoxically served to increase the overall burden of labor on women. These processes are racialized as well as gendered in character; as Kalpana Wilson (2015:807) explains, the production of "hyper-industrious, altruistic, entrepreneurial female subjects" in neoliberal development discourse is bound up with the expansion and intensification of women's labor across the Global South, as a central strategy of capital accumulation.

This evidence draws attention to the increasingly powerful role of transnational governance actors such as the World Bank and the IMF in restructuring the organization of social reproduction in the Global South. It also illuminates the political economic logics and imperatives that underpin development interventions on women's empowerment, particularly when contextualized within the World Bank's "gender equality as smart economics" framework (Roberts and Soederberg 2012) and broader trends of upscaling civil society and downscaling state provisioning. Of particular relevance to this chapter is how empowerment approaches premised on voluntarism have contradictory and/or negative impacts on existing gender and sexual power relations and the distribution of (re)productive labor and how this works to reinforce class relations and hierarchies of gender, sexuality, and race. To date, however, scant attention has been paid to these dynamics in the context of development interventions on HIV and peer education amongst MSM. In light of this, I now turn to the main issues raised by current and former peer educators regarding the operation of peer education programs: first, financial compensation.

ISSUES OF FINANCIAL COMPENSATION

All the peer educators I interviewed in Ghana stated that the money offered to them by NGOs engaged in peer education was insufficient, not just in comparison to a proper wage that would cover living costs, but to meet the basic expenses arising from the work, such as travel, condom distribution, and testing and counseling. As indicated in the standard operating procedures, rather than providing condoms and lubricant for free, peer educators are expected to sell these items to their peers, since it is envisaged that the financial investment, however small, will act as an incentive for the men to use them. In order to do this, peer educators buy the condoms beforehand from the NGO, which, along with other expenses such as travel, significantly eats into their stipend. These practices evoke what Alan Ingram (2012:438) calls "entrepreneurial rationalities" in the global HIV response, that is, the ways in which market logics are legitimated through a neoliberal "discourse of scarcity." In the Ghanaian context, these logics are both embedded in and reproductive of the material conditions in which peer education programs are implemented. As Adam noted, often peers do not have any money to pay for condoms or for the STI or HIV testing services they are encouraged to use. In these situations, many peer educators end up paying out for these items and services out of their own pockets:

> For those with HIV, they are not living. So I talk to them, I counsel them, I pay their hospital folders, even consultation fees to see doctors. I pay it with my own money.

Both during his time as a peer educator and since leaving his role, Adam has sought to provide material (and emotional) support to queer men who are affected by HIV and other STIs. In a seemingly intentional reversal of the preferred public health term "person living with HIV," he described these men's lives as bereft of meaning and vitality—alive but not alive—a situation that he has attempted to counter by giving money toward medical fees and by offering counseling.

As well as financial concerns, peer educators noted that they are often required to work longer hours than officially recognized, as their responsibilities are considerably more time-consuming than accounted for. The standard operating procedures do not stipulate an exact amount of hours peer educators are expected to work; in practice this depends on how quickly and effectively the men realize their quotas. Peer educators' extensive official (and unofficial) responsibilities, combined with the lack of adequate financial remuneration, had prompted a number of research participants to leave peer education. As in Adam's case, this was not because they intended to stop activism altogether, but reflected growing anger over the terms and conditions of their involvement in peer education work and with local, national, and global development organizations. The fact that many of these men continued with other types of community activism, which is in itself both voluntary and unpaid, suggests that the issue was not exclusively or essentially about financial reward, but a question of compensation, recognition, and "who benefits."

ISSUES OF RECOGNITION

Even among long-standing community activists working in peer education, issues of financial compensation engendered a great deal of anger and resentment. Community activists pointed out that they were carrying out some of the most difficult, dangerous, and time-consuming aspects of development organizations' work on MSM and sexual health rights in Ghana, while at the same time failing to benefit from or to be appropriately recognized for their contributions. In the quotation that begins this chapter, Marcus, a former peer educator, explains that peer education is challenging, skilled, and requires dedication, and is fundamentally different from the "office work" of NGOs. Marcus's comment, "You have to always be there," parallels Adam's description of the support he offers to queer men in his community and sheds further light on the onerous and emotionally demanding character of peer education work and community activism in general.

The contrast Marcus draws between the office and report-writing activities of NGOs and the "pure practical work" of peer education illustrates the powerful sense of difference that exists between peer educators and NGO staff. Given the myriad duties, metrics, and monitoring and evaluation procedures that MSM peer educators are expected to follow and fulfill, this is perhaps not surprising. Yet anger over the symbolic and material status of NGO staff among peer educators also reveals how inequalities are (re)produced through health-dominated development agendas and funding regimes. These processes and practices prioritize an NGO-ized "professional technocratic approach" over a more political, grassroots one (Tsikata 2009:186). They also work to co-opt some professional civil society actors into the structures of global governance, while excluding and/or marginalizing other, potentially more radical actors. This co-optation can be understood as part of the broader processes through which neoliberal development interventions have facilitated the exploitation of certain forms of gendered and racialized labor across the Global South: in this context, this includes the *sexualized* social reproductive labor of queer working-class men.

According to my interlocuters, it was not just the scale and scope of queer men's involvement in peer education, and the dedication this requires, that made the work so difficult. By engaging in very visible forms of outreach—which often extended beyond the original remit of HIV and sexual health rights education—peer educators also found themselves at increased risk of homophobic violence and stigmatization. These dynamics parallel findings in Malawi, which indicate that peer educators may be "mocked, attacked, or presumed to be gay amid widespread homophobia" (Biruk and Trapence 2017:343). As Gabriel and Adam explained:

> GABRIEL: Sometimes we, the peer educators, go [to the community] and they beat us.
>
> ADAM: Yes, they will beat us. They don't understand us. They say, "You are teaching people how to do MSM."

Here Gabriel and Adam describe being physically attacked by community members who suspect that they were seeking to "promote" homosexuality through their peer education activities. These dangers were further highlighted by Richie, one of the youngest activists I met, who shared the experience of a peer educator who committed suicide following a homophobic attack:

> May his soul rest in perfect peace . . . He went for outreach and he was doing education and then this group of guys just barged into the room and started beating him, saying, "Gay." They could see the penis model, condom, everything.

Richie contextualized this story by explaining that the peer educator had already "been through so much." In Richie's view, it was the cumulative effect of his colleague's experiences of violence and homophobia that led him to take his own life. Nonetheless, as this story demonstrates so heartbreakingly, peer education work entails a great deal of personal risk for the men involved, not least because of the visibility it brings to them and to the groups of queer men they gather together in the community. This reveals how homophobia not only shapes and reconfigures activists' political activities in an organizational sense, as seen in the case study of CEPEHRG in Chapter 2, but has very material, violent, and occasionally tragic consequences for queer men engaged in sexual health rights work.

Finally, many peer educators that I interviewed noted that carrying penis models, condoms, and lubricant—the mobile tool-kit of a peer educator—is risky and attracts attention, as does wearing the branded T-shirts supplied by funders to identify them as peer educators. Some men explained that they had explicitly requested *not* to wear branded T-shirts on the grounds of safety. Their requests were refused, however, by NGO staff, who told them this was a key criterion of the funding and therefore the project's implementation. This is what Biruk and Trapence (2017:340) term navigating the "economy of harms" associated with peer education-based community engagement, that is, "a network of social relations that hinge on transactions and obligations that are simultaneously risky and potentially profitable." In the Ghanaian context, HIV/LGBTI organizations have been drawn into this economy of harms through processes of NGO-ization. Their response to peer educators' fears over safety thus reflects the managerialist logics that have permeated the organizational culture of the NGO and the ways in which top-down and at times hierarchical management practices are adopted by implementing partners. It also demonstrates the extent to which smaller NGOs—who are operating in the context of increasingly stringent funding conditions—fear losing donor monies or patronage for not following the rules of the game, even where this puts their intended beneficiaries and workers at risk of physical harm. These dynamics indicate that development funding arrangements premised on fixed, quantifiable targets and outcomes and upward-facing reporting and accountability mechanisms are insensitive to the contexts in which activists are working. Moreover, they serve to reinforce rather than unsettle existing divides and power asymmetries, in this context, between the more middle-class sphere of Ghanaian civil society and working-class community networks (and in some instances make them worse, by increasing queer individuals' risk of homophobic violence or abuse). The divisive impacts of peer education programs and the extent of disillusionment and anger peer educators seriously undermine the credibility of these interventions' claims to "community empowerment."

ISSUES OF REPRESENTATION AND ACCOUNTABILITY

Another key source of contention among research participants was the discrepancy between the salaries of NGO workers and their volunteer allowances. This feeling of inequality was compounded both by the sense that working-class queer men are undertaking the most difficult aspects of this work and are not being sufficiently compensated for their efforts, as described above, and by the lack of representation from queer individuals within the organizations themselves. Almost all of the peer educators I met were critical of the lack of representation from and accountability toward working-class queer communities within the NGOs engaged with HIV and LGBTI rights work in Ghana. This finding parallels Dzodzi Tsikata's critique of the impact of neoliberal development agendas, both national and global, on women's organizations in Ghana, which she argues are characterized by a "lack of a mass base, connection and accountability" (2009:186). As Roger Koranteng, a former peer educator with CEPEHRG, explained:

> In Ghana, LGBTI organizations are not accountable to the LGBTI communities. Organizations working for the community should be ready to be accountable to the community: "This is what we use the money for. This is how you are involved. These are the reports. This is what happened." When it happens that way, then it is a fifty-fifty job. You are accountable to us and we help you do this.

In this excerpt, Roger raises the issue of financial as well as programmatic accountability, an allusion that reflects broader suspicions among peer educators and other community activists as to where and how development funds for MSM and sexual rights are being used in Ghana. Anthony Mireku, another former peer educator, explained further:

> Funders and donors always give money to people who are not really doing the work but just sit in their offices. They write big, big reports about MSM and then they collect monies from them. Monies go into the wrong hands and there is mismanagement.

Anthony's comment that "they are not really doing the work" reflects the feeling that activists are, at best, being inadequately recognized for and, at worst, being exploited by their involvement in peer education work. For Anthony, it is the NGOs writing "big, big reports" that claim recognition and financial reward for peer educators' work and activism from donors, while at the same time mismanaging and misdirecting funds away from the intended beneficiaries.

Concerns over financial and programmatic mismanagement were echoed by many other peer educators and community activists and were frequently tied to criticisms of the lack of representation and participation from queer men and the wider "LGBTI community" within NGOs. As Frankie, another former peer educator noted, "Things for the people must be done by the people." Frankie's comment reflects the importance activists attach to the rights to self-determination and self-organization, a sentiment that has caused a small number of the activists I met to leave peer education and sexual health rights work in Accra in order to start up their own independent, community-focused queer and LGBTI groups.

PEER EDUCATION AS SOCIAL REPRODUCTION

Whereas feminist scholars of development have largely focused on women's contribution to social reproduction, this analysis suggests that these processes and activities are incorporating the unpaid labor of other subordinate subjectivities, namely working-class queer men. In the Global North, studies have scarcely examined queer men's contribution to social reproduction (Andrucki 2017), except in relation to domesticity and homemaking (Cook 2014; Pilkey 2014; Vider 2014) or, from a more materialist perspective, by looking at (middle class) gay men's role as consumers (Hennessy 2000, 2006). Nonetheless, there are obvious parallels with the ways in which some gay and lesbian communities in Europe and the United States—although not necessarily framed in terms of social reproduction in the literature—played a critical role in providing care and support to those affected by the AIDS crisis during the 1980s, in the face of lacking institutional response and state indifference (Shephard 1997; Weeks 2000). Many Ghanaian peer educators similarly report that their work encompasses community aftercare, support, and informal caring for men diagnosed and living with HIV, in addition to the activities detailed in their job description relating to health promotion and prevention. Moreover, the combination of extremely limited resources and structural barriers to treatment means that this work is frequently emotionally challenging and at times distressing, an issue that was raised again and again by those involved in HIV work in Accra.[8] Mawuli Gbekor, for example, explained the round-the-clock support he provided to a queer friend who had recently been diagnosed with HIV:

> If I have anything doing, I have to make sure I'm always with him. If he calls and there is any difficulty, I have to rush to him, wherever I am. Even if I have to travel, I make sure that we visit the clinic before I go.

One key difference to the Euro-American situation in the 1980s is that, in the context of MSM interventions, queer men are being formally co-opted into these programs by key policy and civil society stakeholders actors at local, national, and international levels (and that considerable development funding has been channeled into this approach): in other words, peer education is a widely adopted policy and programmatic priority. As in the case of women's work, then, there is theoretical, empirical, and political urgency in rendering visible this type of devalued reproductive labor, especially in Africa, where the everyday, caring, and affective practices of queer individuals have been historically overlooked and where queer people continue to face multiple forms of oppression and exploitation.

CONCLUSION

This chapter has sought to bring insights from the feminist political economy literature on social reproduction and women's empowerment approaches in development to bear on the experiences of MSM peer educators in Ghana. By centring forms of social reproductive labor among queer men in Africa (i.e., as opposed to the extant literature's predominant focus on women and gendered forms of labor) and illuminating how this is mobilized and co-opted by the global development industry, the analysis provides new insights into the everyday political economy of the global HIV response. It also illuminates how this is shaped by neoliberal rationalities and the imperatives of social reproduction in the context of crisis.

At a more practical level, the experiences of former and current peer educators in Ghana raise serious questions about how HIV prevention programs are operationalized in parts of Africa, particularly in terms of their reliance on unpaid caring labor, their effectiveness in relation to supposed empowerment objectives, and the divisive impact they have on existing formations of queer politics. My intention here has not been to attribute responsibility for these dynamics to the small number of NGOs involved in frontline HIV and LGBTI rights work in Ghana. Rather, peer educators and other community activists' frustration with existing HIV/LGBTI organizations reflects the limitations of sexual health rights approaches, how development processes work through (and reproduce) existing inequalities, including inadequate state provisioning for basic needs and the uneven distribution of resources, and the negative consequences of NGO-ization for political activism in this setting. Put more simply, in a context where LGBTI/HIV organizations compete for a highly circumscribed set of funding opportunities, attempt to reshape their organizational priorities in order to fit pre-established development agendas, and are subject to top-down, bureaucratic, and frequently unrealistic management and performance targets, they struggle to connect with the concerns and needs of working-class queer communities.

By examining in detail queer men's experiences of peer education work in Ghana, this chapter has also drawn attention to shifts in the global governance of development and examined what this means for relations of social reproduction, against the backdrop of the HIV epidemic. In so doing, it has shed new light into the types of (gendered, racialized, territorialized, and sexualized) caregiving labor (and laborers) on which the social reproduction of the global economy relies. The contingent, contradictory, and, as I have argued, exploitative ways in which MSM are incorporated into the global HIV response shows how queer bodies and labor are, like women's bodies and labor, effectively acting as "shock absorbers" in the crises of social reproduction characteristic of the neoliberal era. While the contribution of MSM peer educators to this type of caring labor may be globally relatively small, in the context of a health emergency like the HIV epidemic, it plays a critical role in tackling the effects and spread of the disease (and maintaining the health of the working-age population). This has important implications for understanding the everyday political economy of HIV prevention, as well as the relationship between social reproduction and the global governance of health more broadly.

While it is important to acknowledge that some peer educators described their involvement with organizations like CEPEHRG as valuable, in terms of building knowledge of sexual and reproductive health and human rights and forging networks of support and connection, these interventions have impacted the practices of resistance taken up by queer activists and organizations in complex ways, not least by engendering division between formal and informal spheres of activism. Understanding this requires us to look beyond the individual-level impacts of peer education and to consider how this model is entangled in (and shaped by) hegemonic development processes, neoliberal market logics, and structures of heteronormativity. Viewed in this light, peer education among MSM constitutes both a form of social reproductive labor that is legitimated through neoliberal discourses of empowerment *and* a development model that reinvests in a primarily biomedical/behavioral approach to HIV prevention. I explore some of the consequences of this approach in detail in the next chapter.

CHAPTER 4

Queer Ghanaian Politics beyond Sexual Health

Quartey suggested we meet at a breezy rooftop bar in Adabraka, an area of central Accra bordering the busy business districts of Makola and Osu. It was Thursday afternoon and the place was deserted. Quartey was waiting for me when I arrived, sipping a bottle of Malt and sorting through some paperwork. His job as an HIV outreach officer at a small sexual health clinic kept him extremely busy, he told me, and this was the first time he had taken a break all week. Quartey had been working in the field of MSM health for nearly ten years and, like many of the men I met, started off his career as a peer educator. He doesn't see himself as an activist, he explained, but as an advocate and support worker for LGBTI communities in Ghana. During our interview, Quartey spoke passionately about issues of MSM and LGBTI rights. Yet he also grappled with the very painful and emotionally difficult aspects of life as a queer person in Ghana, explaining in frank terms how he tried to cope with what he called his "dual life."

Quartey first experienced sexual desire for other men when he was around fourteen years old. Feeling guilty and ashamed, he tried to keep his feelings secret, swearing to himself that he would never act on his desires. By the time he was eighteen, Quartey was finding it harder and harder to repress his sexuality. Increasingly, he told me, he sought solace in the teachings and practices of the church: "It came to a time I wanted to surrender life to Christ. I wanted to denounce my sexuality." Having confided in a mentor from his congregation, the two of them embarked on a program of prayer and fasting in a bid to cure Quartey of his homosexuality. "We pray, we pray, and we fast. We pray, we fast," he explained, "for days at a time." Despite his efforts, his feelings remained the same. "But it still didn't work," Quartey explained, laughing softly. "Nothing. So I realized naturally maybe that's how I am. I'm born this way."

In some ways, Quartey's attempts to cure himself of his feelings for other men have helped him to come to terms with his sexual orientation: "And I will keep saying I was born this way. There is no way I can change it unless God changes me. I can't change myself." Throughout our interview, however, Quartey returned to the topic of transformation, repeatedly emphasizing his intention to change his lifestyle and behaviors. In this sense, Quartey was very open about his struggle to accept his feelings for men and his desire to give up queer life.

One key consideration for Quartey was his family and his mother in particular. Quartey's father left when he was three, leaving his mother to bring him up on her own. They are, he said, very close. Quartey thinks his mother found out about his sexual orientation from one of his cousins. They have spoken about it candidly and at some length. Although difficult for her to understand, Quartey said, she has accepted it for the time being, as long as he promises to give her a grandchild. "In our culture, if you are a man, you should bear children for your parents," he explained. Quartey's shoulders dropped as he said this, and it was clear that the burden of his mother's expectations weighed heavily. "As an only child, my mum is still expecting a child. At least I should have a child for her."

Later in the interview, I asked Quartey what makes him happy. He told me: "It's when we all gather together, a party, a social gathering, and we are all fooling around. And we have our freedom and we are doing things together. It's so sweet. But when you come back home, you should be the straight boy and the pretender."

Quartey emphasized the multiplicity and, in a sense, duplicity of queer life, the pleasure—the "sweetness"[1]—of queer social events and parties, and the difficulties of coming home to be "the straight boy and the pretender." Because of his sexual orientation, Quartey was constantly forced to be different people in different contexts: he continued, "We're always changing faces. Today we are like that and tomorrow we are here, we are like that." These are not queer becomings in the sense of playful articulations of difference, but rather the difficult, compromised negotiations made by someone who is caught between hegemonic power structures and norms: between familial pressures, expectations of heterosexuality, marriage, and fatherhood.

At the end of our interview, I asked Quartey about his hopes and fears for the future. Again, he returned to his desire to renounce the *sasso* lifestyle, to "stop being gay," as he put it. "I see myself maybe married, having children, and saying goodbye to such a lifestyle. Becoming a better person." Quartey's emphasis on having children supports what Akosua Adomako Ampofo (2009) terms the centrality of "phallic competence"—that is, of biological reproduction—to constructs of masculinity in Ghana. Despite his work advocating for sexual health rights for MSM, Quartey wished he could fulfill his mother's expectations and live what he called "a better life." He concluded, "You can't be gay throughout your life. You need to get married one day. You need to have children one day."

Quartey's story captures some of the tensions between resistance and accommodation, defiance and conformity that characterize queer lived experience in Ghana, including within the field of sexual health rights advocacy. While by no means universal, Quartey's feelings about his sexual orientation and hopes for the future find parallels in the stories of many of the men I met who were engaged in HIV prevention activities among MSM. It is the apparent irreconcilability of his dual lives and desires, as Quartey described it, that is particularly striking. This irreconcilability reveals something important about the ways in which the selective conceptualization of rights—and individualized understandings of change—that are embedded in sexual health approaches resonate with, and at times reinforce, experiences of homophobia and oppression in Ghana. In Quartey's case, his work for an NGO led him away from more community-based forms of resistance and, it seems, has done little to resolve his personal struggle with self-acceptance. Faced with the daily realities of the HIV epidemic and queer men's poor health outcomes in his work, and with the seeming impossibility of queerness in his home life, it is understandable that Quartey should feel that things would simply be easier if he were straight.

THE LANDSCAPE OF QUEER STRUGGLE IN GHANA

Legal repression, discrimination, homophobia, and violence profoundly limit the life outcomes of queer working-class Ghanaians. As some of the stories included in this book demonstrate, visibly, publicly, or indeed reputedly queer Ghanaian men struggle to find stable work and housing, are rejected by family and friends, and are more likely to engage in sex work and other transactional sexual relations. This, in turn, shapes their disproportionate vulnerability to HIV, alcohol and substance abuse, ill health, and, ultimately, premature death. Since beginning my research into HIV and LGBTI rights activism in Ghana in the early 2010s, a number of the men I met have experienced deteriorating physical and mental health, battles with addiction and substance misuse, and complex medical crises. Tragically, several of them have passed away. As Kobby Mensah, from Maritime Life Precious Foundation, highlighted, the consequences of queer oppression are far-reaching and are not being adequately addressed through existing sexual health interventions:

> In Ghana we are only seeing the issue of MSM through the window of HIV. All the donor efforts and resources are channeled into getting results for HIV outcomes. But you have to recognize that there are so many issues we are facing. I've told people from USAID, 'there are other things that need to be addressed.' But you find that you can only talk to them about health.

Scholarship on LGBTI activism in Africa has documented the strategic advantages and disadvantages of adopting less visible, more discrete, public health approaches to LGBTI rights (Epprecht 2011, 2013; Currier 2012; Currier and McKay 2017). This chapter argues that rather than having pros and cons, public health approaches fail to recognize and tackle the structural drivers of queer oppression and, in so doing, sideline other more radical—and potentially transformative—agendas and activities among working-class queer communities. To advance this argument, the chapter explores four priorities for queer struggle as identified in the narrative testimonies and everyday practices of queer activists and community networks in Accra, namely: improving mental health and well-being, preventing homophobic violence, tackling poverty, and finding decent work.[2] While a lack of legal LGBTI rights and protections is a key part of this—particularly in terms of discrimination—queer liberation is understood as a struggle for economic as well as erotic justice: it is about addressing unemployment, low incomes, poverty, precarity, and class inequality. The chapter demonstrates that only by paying closer attention to the everyday political economy of queer oppression and resistance can we fully understand the limitations of prevailing development agendas and policies: in simple terms, why sexual health rights are not enough.

The chapter begins by elucidating how sexual health interventions—which organize queer individuals around an agenda of risk, vulnerability, and disease prevention—resonate with activists' experiences of homophobia, shaping understanding of embodiment, gender expression, and desire, and ultimately, reinforcing heterosexist norms. I contextualize this in relation to widespread homophobic violence in Ghana and show why addressing violence and improving standards of living are such key issues for working-class queer activists. This analysis further illuminates the regressive consequences of selective, partial, and health-oriented approaches to LGBTI rights and how they work to depoliticize and individualize struggle. In the second part of the chapter, I examine the landscape and horizons of queer Ghanaian activism beyond the purview of development and sexual health. This analysis shows how queer individuals and networks are resisting and pushing back against homophobia at a grassroots level, on the issues that are important to them. They do so through four primary activities: queer kinship practices, claiming and queering space, community conflict mediation, and legal rights claims. These everyday practices and modes of organizing address, on their own terms and in their own ways, the priorities for struggle set out above. Accordingly, they hold important insights for understanding the character of queer oppression and resistance in Ghana and for external actors seeking to defend, promote, and support LGBTI rights in the country.

CHANGING BEHAVIOR, REINFORCING NORMS

Before examining the political priorities of queer community activists in detail, I wish to reflect a little on Quartey's preoccupation with transformation and on the psychological effects of queer men's engagement in HIV and sexual health promotion work for NGOs. While Chapter 3 examined the implications of peer education initiatives from the perspective of labor and social reproduction, this chapter examines their more embodied and ideational consequences. "Behavior change" is one of the founding principles of HIV prevention and refers to a set of behavioral measures that aim to reduce the risk of contracting HIV, namely condom usage, partner reduction, and reduction of other "risky" sexual practices. In Ghana, however, the concept has taken on a new meaning among some LGBTI/HIV organizations and their staff, namely to describe the ways in which queer men can modify dissident gender expression to align more closely with normative ideas of masculinity.

The following excerpt comes from a group interview conducted with three former and current peer educators in Jamestown, an area of central Accra, in which the participants described the personal processes of behavior change that have resulted from their involvement in HIV prevention work:

ELLIE: Do you think, since you were teenagers, there have been any changes in attitudes toward homosexuality?

P3: We have changed.

P2: Yes . . . at first, the kind of dress that we put on.

P3: [Interrupting]—the way we behave.

P2: The kind of way we behave, the way we walk.

P3: The way we put on eye shadow.

P2: At first we used to put on ladies' cloth.

P3: We wear ladies' cloth and things because you want people to see you, like, that is you, that is you, that is you. But . . .

P1: But now behavior change.

P2: Yes, behavior change.

The participants discuss modifying practices such as wearing women's clothes and putting on makeup, as well as changing certain mannerisms, such as how they walk. I asked participants about the motivation for this type of behavior change, which represents a clear departure from the original public health concept. According to Gabriel Quaye, a peer educator with CEPEHRG, it was mainly about safety for the organizations leading MSM peer education programs in Accra:

> It's because people will wear feminine dress to the office and people will recognize that this is what the office is doing. At first the organization was at Osu, but they had to move from one place to another. And then getting to another place, they don't want the MSM to come and spoil the community for them. So you have to dress sharp, as a guy.

Gabriel's suggestion that MSM will come and "spoil the community" evokes a pathological view of MSM and gender non-conformity in particular, in the same way that his argument that you have to "dress sharp like a guy" values the sartorial scripts of hegemonic masculinity over practices of queer bodily transgression. A number of peer educators also explained that they had started going to the gym and lifting weights as a means to better protect themselves from homophobic violence, a strategy they advised should be adopted by other feminine-presenting queer men. This very physical process of transformation, although understandable in terms of safety, works to reproduce and reinforce normative constructions of masculinity (as well as marginalizing others), here in terms of dress, mannerisms, and physique. The importance of this kind of behavior change was also highlighted by Adam:

> Behavior change means you shouldn't dress very effeminate, you shouldn't wear skirts, you shouldn't wear tight stuffs and be skirmishing around.[3] Because if you do that, there are people around who will think you are [sasso], and they will know you are vulnerable.

Antieffeminacy in gay male culture has been observed across a number of geographic settings in the Global North (Taywaditep 2002; Sánchez et al. 2016; Sánchez and Vilian 2012). It is a phenomenon that is understood to be related to men's negative feelings about being gay and factors such as the difficulty of coming out. Such explanations are potentially germane in Ghana, given the risks to physical safety entailed in being publicly out and evidence of internalized homophobia among African MSM communities (Kushwaha et al. 2017). For Quartey, however, behavior change is not only about processes of defeminization, or modifying dissident gender expression, but extends to other aspects of queer men's lifestyles, including their speech, public perceptions, and work aspirations. As Quartey explained:

> So far as in African settings, no matter how 100 percent you are in the LGBTI community, you would sometimes have to confront other members of the society. So it is important for people to have a bit of change in mind: how they dress, how they talk, how seriously they take their career.

Quartey's concerns about safety are again imbued with normative ideas of masculinity—as in the suggestion that queer men should change "how they dress, how they talk"—as well as more moralistic (and aspirational) notions of appropriate behavior, as in the suggestion that queer men have to "take their career seriously." In this sense, behavior change is not just a pragmatic strategy taken up by some LGBTI/HIV organizations and peer educators to negotiate homophobic violence or manage issues of visibility, but is used in more internalized, normative, and disciplinary ways. Zachary Nortey, for example, another former peer educator, highlighted the stigma attached to gender nonconformity in Ghana, but for him, the problem lies with feminine-presenting men themselves for "attracting attention." He explained: "The people I think have had a very bad impact is the same gay guys who behave girlish. Anywhere you will be that they will come, they will attract attention."

The negativity some queer men display toward gender nonconformity and feminine gender expression in particular is encapsulated in the Twi phrase *ɔbaa pe kyɛ*. Meaning literally in English "soft or weak woman," this description, I was told, could be used to refer to a queer man whose mannerisms are perceived to be too feminine in character.

These expanded and refashioned interpretations of behavior change were not one-off remarks or idiosyncrasies, but were referenced frequently and consistently by many of the current and former peer educators and NGO-based activists I met and interviewed. This shows how individual-level, biomedical warnings about risk, danger, and HIV—and the broader strategy of medicalizing queer sexualities in development—refract through localized gender hierarchies and forms of homophobia to (re)shape queer men's feelings about their own sexual orientations and gender expressions. In the case of individuals like Quartey and Zachary, it shores up a hegemonic view of what is means to be a man in Ghana, as well as internalized negativity toward feminine gender presentation and forms of transgressive gendered embodiment. In so doing, it has a depoliticizing and deradicalizing effect; it reinforces heterosexist norms, creates an individualized sense of responsibility, and promotes a view of the individual (and specifically the person's behavior) as the key agent of change and locus of power.

Some readers may question what queer men's understandings of embodiment and the self have to do with development or political economy. But Quartey's and the other men's stories powerfully illuminate the workings of heteronormativity in Ghana and how development interventions can bolster hegemonic social and economic power relations and norms. In the context of HIV prevention initiatives, neoliberal economic rationalities produce MSM as sociosexual subjects: autonomous, individualized, responsibilized (Kapileni et al. 2004; Kerr and Mkandawire 2012; see also Griffin 2007). These dynamics—autonomization, individualization, responsibilization—conceal the role of structural factors in producing health inequalities and place the onus on the individual (rather than, for example, the state) to address their causes and effects. They also contribute to a wider process of material-discursive interpellation that not only renders queer men individually responsible for their health and well-being, but embeds a logic that permeates many other areas of their life: professional, familial, financial, erotic. As Wendy Brown (2003) argues, the penetration of economic rationalities into formerly noneconomic domains "prescribes citizen-subject conduct in a neo-liberal order." This means that neoliberalism is a political rationality that shapes and governs *behavior*, rather than just a particular mode of state-market relations or set of economic policy prescriptions. In this instance, these rationalities are operating through biomedical technologies intended to manage HIV risk and vulnerability.

At a more symbolic level, privileging the sexual and epidemiological aspects of queer men's lives lends credence to the idea that gay men are "vectors" of disease and to the pathological representations of homosexuality found within mainstream Ghanaian media. Evidently, the incendiary and misleading reporting of some media outlets is not the fault of Ghana's LGBTI/HIV organizations and, as CEPEHRG's experiences of backlash highlight, questions of visibility, resistance, and confrontation are extremely fraught in the context of intense (and intensifying) politicization. Yet the confluence of disease-related, medicalized conceptualizations of queer sexuality in development and homophobic political discourse is given a particular kind of power in the absence of more positive, affirmative, or radical articulations of rights and justice from prominent organizational actors. In this analysis, I am particularly concerned with the effects of this approach on queer men themselves: as demonstrated in the refashioning of the concept of behavior change, sexual health initiatives are engendering complex psychological responses among the men with which they engage, in relation to their own struggles with homophobia and norms of masculinity. This is especially problematic given the broader mental health impacts of homophobia and oppression in Ghana.

THE PUBLIC AND PRIVATE TERRAIN OF HOMOPHOBIC VIOLENCE

Homophobic violence, widely documented across parts of southern and East Africa (Reid and Dirsuweit 2002; Mkhize et al. 2010; Msibi 2016), is an endemic feature of queer working-class life in Ghana. Navigating public space normatively coded as heterosexual, visibly queer individuals are at high risk of physical or verbal abuse, threats, and assault. Many of these cases are not reported to the authorities and reliable data on the scale of homophobically motivated violence in Ghana are not available. Nonetheless, a number of incidents have received mainstream media attention in the country over the past decade. This includes a violent assault on a lesbian couple in Accra in 2012 (VibeGhana 2012), a gang attack on a suspected gay marriage ceremony in Jamestown in 2012 (Okertchiri 2012), gatherings of "anti-gay mobs" in Tamale in March 2013 (Daily Guide 2013), and an attempted lynching of two women accused of lesbianism by a gang of youths in Kumasi in 2018 (Nettey 2018), to name just a few. During one of my research visits to Ghana in 2015, a man suspected of being gay was subjected to a particularly brutal assault in the Nima area of Accra by a vigilante group called "Safety Empire" (see *Daily Guide* 2015b). Although these kind of attacks occur with alarming frequency, the brutality of the Nima assault sent shockwaves through the city's close-knit network of activists.

Media reports of homophobic violence are borne out in the stories of many queer men I interviewed in Accra. The 2013 gang attack on a queer party in Jamestown was referred to often, not least because the area was believed to be relatively queer-friendly, as compared to other parts of the city, prior to the incident.[4] It is obviously difficult to establish a causal link between the politicization of homosexuality over the past twenty years and specific incidents of homophobic violence. But for many activists there is little doubt that the increasingly hostile climate surrounding homosexuality, particularly as this is fueled by newspaper, TV, and radio reports, has intensified queer individuals' vulnerability to violence and abuse. Attitudinal surveys conducted over the last decade give some sense of the scale of negativity toward homosexuality among the general population in Ghana; according to a Pew Research Center study conducted in 2013, 96 percent of Ghanaians agree with the statement "homosexuality should not be accepted by society" (Pew Research Center 2013:1). In 2014, another Pew study found that 98 percent of the Ghanaian population view homosexuality as "morally unacceptable," the highest percentage score among forty countries surveyed (Pew Research Center 2014:5).

Homophobic violence extends beyond the public sphere into the private, with interview participants recounting experiences of intimate partner violence, as well as frequent violence at the hands of family members, relatives, neighbors, or even friends. Studies of heterosexual violence in Ghana find that patriarchal gender norms and intrahousehold power inequalities underpin and contexualize patterns of violence (Mann and Takyi 2009; Takyi and Mann 2006), particularly between husbands and wives. In the context of homophobic violence, it is a specifically heterosexist construct of masculinity—predicated on heterosexual sexual orientation and masculine gender presentation—that is being policed and enforced (Epprecht 2004). One young activist and former peer educator, Ziggy Laryea, was asleep in bed when his mother's boyfriend entered into his room and violently beat him, breaking his leg. Although the boyfriend was drunk and they had argued previously, Ziggy did not see the attack coming. According to him, it was motivated by his "effeminate" mannerisms and tendency to wear earrings and makeup. Ziggy was eventually thrown out of the family home and forced to take a room in a shared compound house in another part of the city. Things had become easier for him, he said, since he stopped dressing so effeminately, wearing tight-fitting clothes, and putting on earrings. Ziggy framed this as a kind of maturing, a growing up, and, in another reference to HIV terminology, as a realization of "behavior change." Ziggy's experiences illustrate the violent sanctions that arise from transgressive forms of gendered embodiment, including in the most intimate of spaces, as well as the ways in which epidemiological concepts of behavior change have been reinterpreted by some peer educators and activists. His experiences also shed light into the complex of class and sexuality in this setting; faced with violence, familial rejection, precarious housing, and a lack of stable employment, Ziggy simply could not risk further transgressing norms of masculinity. His priority at the moment, he told me during our interview, was maintaining his rent and building the small business he had started selling food.

HOMOPHOBIA AND MENTAL HEALTH

The mental health impacts of homophobia among queer African men have begun to attract attention in the public health literature, notably in relation to how internalized homophobia limits access to HIV testing and treatment (Adebajo et al. 2012) and, geographically, in the context of southern Africa (Cook et al. 2013; see also Müller and Daskilewicz 2018).[5] This forms part of a wider body of scholarship that documents the links between structural factors, such as unemployment, poverty, criminalization, and discrimination, and psychosocial factors, such as self-stigmatization and internalized homophobia, in shaping and determining vulnerability to HIV. However, less attention has been paid to the nexus of homophobia and poor mental health in the context of LGBTI rights activism in Africa; this is particularly the case when it comes to thinking through how activists conceptualize their priorities for struggle.

Benjamin Yemoh, an activist closely involved in peer education work in Accra, told me that he was shocked by the scale and severity of mental health issues among MSM and among the wider queer community. He explained: "People are dying day in and out. People are taking their own lives because of frustration and depression." During our interview, Benjamin emphasized the mental health impacts of oppression, inequality, and a lack of LGBTI rights and, like many of the other men I spoke to, recounted stories of friends who had attempted suicide or had taken their own lives because of struggles related to their sexual orientation and/or gender expression. A number of interview participants also shared their own personal battles with despair, hopelessness, and thoughts of self-harm.

According to Ike Bentil, a former peer educator and community activist, queer men's struggles with suicidality and feelings of worthlessness are as much about poverty and unemployment, as they are about HIV. This, he pointed out, is what determines the ineffectiveness of HIV interventions that encourage condom usage and other reductions in "risky behaviors":

> When I have job, I have some skills, and there's some respect for my life, then I have a reason to live. And a reason to use condom and lubricant. But when my life is not even worth living, I don't know what I'm living for, there's nothing. . . . That is why the programs are not really helping.

In this way, community activists demonstrate a very clear understanding of the structural roots of inequality and vulnerability, particularly in terms of how material constraints, such as a lack of employment opportunities and discrimination, combine with mental health issues to lead queer men into the types of transactional sexual relations that increase their risk of HIV. As Benjamin explained:

> But if we keep on talking about HIV, we keep on producing the condom without the person working, he moves back and has sex. What do you do when you meet someone who is ready to give you lunch, a chunk of money, and you are not working? And they say, "I won't use condom." You end up risking your life just because you don't have the money.

While many peer educators and community- and NGO-based activists expressed concerns over the limitations of sexual health approaches to LGBTI rights, a small number of activists advocated abandoning NGO-led activism altogether. Francis Tetteh was one of the first men recruited to MSM peer education work in Accra, as part of the SHARP project that began in 2004. He worked as a peer educator for a number of years, but became increasingly unhappy with the terms and conditions of the work, especially the lack of recognition given to, and accountability toward, peer educators. As a result of his experiences, he decided to disconnect himself from Accra's formal LGBTI/HIV organizations and to dedicate his time to more grassroots forms of community building. I met Francis frequently during my research: he was loud and outspoken, always cracking jokes and telling stories, and was well known among the queer networks of central Accra. For Francis, queer activists and organizations must go beyond a single-issue approach to struggle, not least because of the deeply contradictory ways in which this plays out on the ground. He explained:

> That, for me, is the challenge I have with our governments in Africa and with the Ghanaian government. A gay person can be arrested and charged with the sodomy law. And then you go for those Global Fund moneys which are specifically for MSM or gay men to run a program. So the question I ask myself is, "How effective are those programs?" Because a gay man who knows he's been criminalized, who knows there's a law that can get him into trouble, will not be coming to you and saying, "Treat me. Help me."

In contrast to organizations like CEPEHRG and HRAC, Francis argued that tackling the legal and institutional drivers of queer men's oppression, that is, criminalization, is key, as is establishing legal protections for LGBTI individuals; as he put it, "we need a law that recognizes and protects us on the basis of our gender and sexuality in Ghana."

POVERTY, LIVING STANDARDS, AND WORK

As this analysis indicates, the primacy attributed to improving queer men's mental health is intimately related to a number of other political issues, namely homophobic violence, economic hardship and poor standards of living, and unemployment. Given queer men's experiences of violence, insecure housing and homelessness, and the difficulties they encounter finding and holding onto work, it is understandable that these should be identified as the most fundamental political priorities of all. George Tagoe, another community activist involved with CEPEHRG, was especially critical of the adoption of Pride events in Ghana, as in the programs organized by HRAC in 2014, given the economic and security issues facing queer individuals in the country.[6] He explained:

People are dying and we need to save lives first. I mean when you talk about a hierarchy of needs you cannot go and put a sick person on the street to parade. Or a hungry person on the street to parade. We need to first look at their security, how we build them economically before we can think about all these other issues.

George's understanding of security and building people economically encompasses more than just physical health and safety to include how queer individuals meet their basic needs. While he noted the powerful nexus of health issues, poverty, and insecurity, for him the starting point was an economic one. The same point was made by Nii Aryitey, another long-standing peer educator and community activist I interviewed. Expressing his anger at what he described as donors' focus on "HIV, HIV, HIV," Nii noted drily, "a man cannot eat condoms and lube." In this way, former peer educators and community activists roundly rejected the health-first approaches to LGBTI rights advanced by key donor governments and development agencies, and operationalized through Ghana's formal LGBTI/HIV organizations. This programmatic and rhetorical framing is not only at odds with the priorities laid out by queer working-class men, including many former and current peer educators, but with the ways in which queer individuals come together to resist homophobia at the grassroots level. In this context, it is the material dimensions of queer oppression that take center stage, specifically the impacts of violence, homophobia, and economic hardship.

QUEER POLITICS BEYOND THE NGO

So far this book has sought to delineate how development interventions on HIV and NGO-led sexual health rights activities have impacted the landscape of queer politics in Ghana. In this section, I explore the queer political practices and forms of organizing that exist outside of this sphere. Kathleen O'Mara (2013) describes the informal, everyday activities that characterize queer networks in Ghana as "community practices," rather than as examples of activism, per se. This is understandable insofar as these practices do not appear to have an agreed or consistent political agenda, are not necessarily concerned with changing state laws or policies, and do not involve substantial numbers of activists. Instead, they take place in a more ad hoc way, in casual community settings among friends and peers, and encompass a range of activities, from quotidian acts of love and support to the courageous attempts of some activists to seek legal redress. I would argue, however, that in a context where homosexuality is criminalized and queer individuals face multiple forms of oppression, it is impossible to separate the personal or the community from the political. As Armisen notes, reflecting on the role of queer social gatherings in West Africa as a political (and politicizing) space: "Although such gatherings had no explicit political agenda, they were political by nature" (2016:10).

Armisen's idea that the collective actions of marginalized people are "political by nature" is illuminating for this analysis. By claiming space, intervening in circumstances of violence and abuse, and offering material and emotional support, activists are directly confronting homophobia and heteronormativity, in their everyday forms. For the purposes of analysis, I organize these everyday practices of resistance into four key areas: queer kinship arrangements, claiming and queering space, community mediation strategies, and legal rights claims.

"NO FAMILY EXCEPT MY LGBTI FAMILY": QUEER KINSHIP

The creation of queer kinship networks was one of the most common political practices described by queer community activists in Accra. Sometimes groups meet in a queer-friendly "spot" (bar); other times they gather by a friend's food stand or shop or in their homes. Although sizable, these networks are very close-knit, with many of the men complaining about the *kɔkɔnsa* (Twi, "gossip") that goes on within the community. Queer social groups are often loosely structured around neighborhoods, with *sassoi* and other queer individuals coming together to form very localized kinship networks. Although typically neighborhood-oriented, kinship networks are fluid and may comprise changing groups of queer individuals. Some of the groups I met were formed from long-standing friendships, dating back to childhood. Most of them, however, were established much more recently and were marked by transience and change. The transient character of these groups reflects, among other things, the difficulties queer individuals face finding secure housing and employment, their experiences of familial rejection and homelessness, and their encounters with homophobic violence and abuse within their own communities. This means that queer individuals are frequently compelled to move between different houses, geographic areas, and, in some instances, cities. As Evans-Love Quansah explained: "People move from Tamale.[7] They've been sacked from their homes, their communities. There are chiefs there who want to kill them because they are LGBTI people."

Atu Annan, an experienced peer educator and community activist in his late twenties, recounted his own personal story of homelessness and displacement:

> My biggest challenge now is finding accommodation. At the moment I'm homeless. I don't have a place of my own. . . . I'm just with our friends here. But I'm not comfortable with it. It's like he needs his privacy and I'm there all the time.

Atu was thrown out of his family home after being confronted about his sexuality by his mother and admitting that he was in a relationship with a man. He was unemployed, he told me, and unable to find alternative long-term accommodation. For nearly a year, Atu was forced to move between the houses of different queer friends—"my brothers," as he called them—staying on their floors. The support of his queer family was critical in helping Atu to cope with the loneliness and isolation he experienced after being thrown out by his mother, as he commented: "No family apart from my LGBTI family. When it comes to biological family, there's nothing." The situation was, however, very distressing for him: "I'm not comfortable with it," as he put it. These difficulties were compounded by the fact that many of Atu's friends also lived in temporary, cramped, or otherwise unsuitable housing. As a result, Atu was occasionally forced to rely on older, financially better-off boyfriends for support.[8]

Atu's description of the support he received from his LGBTI family sheds light into the character and functions of queer kinship practices in Ghana. One central aspect of these relationships involves the provision of material support when queer kin need help, for example, with accommodation, food, or clothing. Offering money to other queer individuals who may be struggling for work or in need of medical treatment was an equally common practice within queer networks, as was connecting queer friends to moneymaking opportunities, such as short-term jobs.

Adam Amoah's stay with a queer, "*sasso*-friendly" woman during his expulsion from his family home, described in Chapter 3, provides another insight into the role of queer kinship relations. For Adam, his stay with his friend (or "auntie," as he called her) was hugely important, bringing him much needed emotional comfort as well as a roof over his head during a very difficult time. As he put it, "There are people whose words make you happy." The affective importance of this type of kin relationship was emphasized again and again by working-class queer men. Mawuli Gbekor, for example, a former peer educator, described his experiences supporting a queer friend through his diagnosis with HIV:

> So we cried together. We cried together without me even saying anything to him, because we knew each other very well, like brothers. So I put everything aside and I made sure we cried and he cried because that was the journey we had to make.

A little like Adam and his auntie, Mawuli's account reveals the intense emotional connections that are forged between queer individuals in the face of poverty and ill health. Mawuli's comment "that was the journey we had to make" conjures up the idea of a mutual grieving process, an act of affective solidarity between two queer friends or "brothers." This type of queer kinship practice is politically and materially important; it creates a social safety net that is otherwise unavailable to queer working-class communities. At the same time, these practices encompass the emotional and the affective; they are about building community, sharing knowledge, providing counseling, creating bonds of solidarity, and offering physical protection. It is these political micropractices—what I would term alternative modes of queer social reproduction—that community activists described as especially meaningful and transformative, much more than their participation in larger and more obviously political events such IDAHOT and Pride.

CLAIMING AND QUEERING SPACE

Another key political practice among queer community networks involves the creation and inhabitation of queer spaces, such as social events, parties, and gatherings in bars or shops. These spaces may not necessarily be read as queer to an outsider, since they frequently take place in public and communal spaces. Nonetheless, they serve important functions, engendering feelings of belonging and togetherness and acting as a site for collective emotional reflection and catharsis. In this sense, they again form part of the multifaceted ways in which queer individuals seek to deal with the emotional and psychological effects of oppression and homophobia.

During my interview with Ziggy, I asked him about a significant moment from his teenage years. He told me the story of a gang he was part of in Accra, the White Angels, between the ages of fifteen and seventeen. The White Angels were made up of Ziggy and a few of his queer friends, who would get together to dress up in women's clothes, put on fake eyelashes, mascara, and earrings, and attend events in the community:

> We will gather at our friend's place and put on our makeup and our eyelashes and we will be moving from one event to another. We will go to parties, go to weddings, go to dinners, go to funerals.

According to Ziggy, these very public displays of gender transgression received a mixed reaction. While some community members saw the White Angels' performances as entertaining, many were hostile, or even abusive. Ziggy and his friends sought to keep the gang's activities a secret from their families for fear of recrimination. At one wedding party, Ziggy was spotted by an auntie who threatened to expose him to his mother if he did not stop what he was doing. Despite these difficulties, Ziggy continued to be part of the gang, and described their performances as some of the most enjoyable moments of his life. He explained: "At these events, we will dance. We will dance so that we will sweat and there will be sweat all over our body. You know those were such happy moments because we didn't care what anybody will say."

Funerals and weddings are usually sizable and significant community events in Ghana. The presence of noticeably queer or gender-nonconforming groups like the White Angels at these events is, in this sense, a form of spatial queering that is subversive and, at times, risky, particularly, in Ziggy's case, since it put him at risk of discovery by family members. At the same time, this defiance is part of the sense of enjoyment and empowerment that Ziggy derived from these events; as he put it, "Those were such happy moments because we didn't care what anybody will say."

The importance of claiming and queering space was also highlighted by James, another former peer educator, in this instance as a way to forge collective forms of emotional support. James described how the creation of queer social events helped him and his friends to share difficult experiences and to come to terms with some of their past traumas:

> We come together. We become part of this family. People are talking, shedding tears, and I realized at some point we're going through some healing process.

Queer spaces—whether large parties or small gatherings—serve as arenas in which queer men are able to share experiences, to receive and give advice, and to celebrate dissident gender expression and sexual orientation (as well as to meet potential partners and/or form erotic connections): "It's like our own mini-Pride," as one activist put it. For many of the men, these spaces were seen as especially important in easing their own personal struggles with self-acceptance. Kofi Acheampong, another former peer educator, encapsulated this in his description of queer get-togethers:

> We share ideas. We jawjaw. People share their horrible experiences. People share their happiest experiences. We have fun. We dance. We swim. We play football. We play all the local female games. And then we, you know, live like we want to live.

As Kofi's comments indicate, creating and queering space is about more than sexual connection; it is about the quotidian practices that generate lifeworlds beyond the repressive horizons of the present. This brings to mind Muñoz's (2009:1) account of "queer futurity," that is, the idea that queerness describes the *future*, not the present: it imagines "new and better pleasures, other ways of being in the world, and ultimately new worlds."

COMMUNITY MEDIATION AND LEGAL RIGHTS CLAIMS

In addition to queer kinship and spatial queering, a number of community activists I spoke to emphasized the importance of a political practice best described as "community mediation." Essentially, community mediation involves getting a group of queer individuals, community activists, and/or other allies together following an incident of homophobic violence, harassment, or abuse. This group will typically consult with the victim and make some kind of intervention, usually by talking to the assailant or by appealing to the assailant's friends and family members. As Edward explained:

> Usually what will happen is you will go and try and talk to the person. To explain to him how his actions are impacting on the victim, you know, and to ask him to stop. Sometimes you have to go several times. Or sometimes you will have to go to the family [of the perpetrator] and appeal to them to intervene.

Edward noted that the results of these interventions are often mixed, since they rely on appealing to the goodwill or "better side," as he put it, of the perpetrator or their family and since activists do not usually have any organizational (or legal) weight behind them.[9] At the same time, for many community activists, mediation was seen as the only viable option in terms of redress, due to the unnatural carnal knowledge law. As Atu pointed out:

> Even when somebody violates your rights you are scared to go to the police to report because the moment you get there, they will say, 'We know you. You are gay, go away.' They wouldn't even listen to your story . . . It's very disheartening living in a country like that where people's rights are just . . . You are there and you cannot say anything. It's very difficult.

In this context, attempts at community mediation serve an important purpose because many queer men are targeted within their own communities by individuals or groups of individuals who are known to them (and, moreover, community mediation does not require activists or other queer individuals to engage with the police). As Adam explained:

> Oh, it can happen right now. Neighbors. That group of guys on the corner. If I get down right now, those guys can just be calling me, "Batty guy, batty faggot, they fuck you in your ass."

According to my interlocuters, these everyday acts of homophobic abuse (which, on occasion, also involve physical and/or sexual violence, harassment, threats, and blackmail) constitute some of the most disturbing and distressing aspects of life as a queer person in Accra. In such an environment, community mediation represents an important way for community activists and other queer individuals to come together and attempt to mitigate their effects.

In more serious cases of violence, harassment, or blackmail—and depending on the wishes of the victim—community activists have also come together, on occasion, to report the case to the police. This is not conflict mediation, in this instance, but an attempt to claim rights and pursue justice. Since there are no specific legal protections afforded to LGBTI individuals under the Ghanaian constitution, this is most commonly done using the right to privacy or laws pertaining to criminal offenses, such as assault, battery, or blackmail. As described earlier, one high-profile case occurred in March 2012, when queer individuals attending a birthday party in the Jamestown area of Accra were assaulted and forced to flee the area by the "Ga-Mashie Youth for Change," a vigilante group who accused partygoers of conducting a gay marriage ceremony. According to those who were there, the group attacked them with canes and cutlasses, stole items such as phones and money, and forced some of them to strip. In the aftermath of the attack, many of the men who were targeted left their homes out of fear for their safety.

Community activists, led by Francis Tetteh, took the case to the Human Rights Advocacy Center (HRAC), then under the leadership of the human rights lawyer Nana Oye Lithur. Lawyers from HRAC accompanied the group to the police and assisted them in filing a case, which was later referred to the Domestic Violence and Victim Support Unit (DOVVSU). Described by one Ghanaian newspaper as a "Clash over Gay Rights" (Okertchiri 2012), the incident received considerable attention in the national press. When interviewed about her support for the victims, Oye Lithur clarified the position of HRAC: "We believe that they are human beings and every single right that is granted through the constitution, they are equally entitled to." In a reference to the right to privacy, she further added, "For me, what they do behind closed doors is their own business" (Okertchiri 2012).

While the support offered by HRAC and Oye Lithur in particular was welcomed by Francis and his friends, their case led to no arrests, and Francis described being "palmed off" by the victim support officer at DOVVSU:

> We are suffering, we are being beaten. Even in this community, we were chased out from this community.[10] Nobody came to our aid. We went to the police station. After we write our reports and all that, some organizations came. They took reports. But there was no follow-up. We are still being beaten in this community. We don't have peace.

Community activists reported that attempts to bring justice for victims through forms of legal redress were typically unsuccessful and often resulted in further experiences of homophobia and discrimination at the hands of police or other judicial and civil society personnel. In the case of the Ga-Mashie Youth for Change attack, for example, the only people arrested in relation to the incident were some of the men who had attended the party. Francis also contrasts the legal support he received from HRAC for this case with his experiences of other state institutions, such as the government's Commission on Human Rights and Administrative Justice (CHRAJ). Under Mahama's administration, CHRAJ appeared to be adopting a more neutral line on homosexuality, which included setting up an online system for PLHIV and KPs to report human rights abuses. The "Discrimination Reporting System," launched in 2013, invites "any person who believes he/she has experienced discrimination on the basis of HIV status, gender identity or sexual orientation to report an incident through the CHRAJ stigma and discrimination reporting portal." According to a report put together by a group of Ghanaian LGBTI, MSM, and other human rights organizations, however, only sixty-six complaints had been filed through the reporting system between 2013 and 2016, of which twenty-seven were from LGBTI individuals (Yussif et al. 2016:3). No figures were available on how many of these cases had been solved.

While the writers of the report broadly welcomed the reporting system, community activists like Francis remained highly critical and wary of actors like CHRAJ. He explained:

> No one is helping. We help ourselves in the community. We were beaten, we go to CHRAJ. They did not look at our face. They see us to be animals. They didn't even talk to us. It was very, very painful. It hurts. But we help ourselves.

Francis's comment that "no one is helping" reflects his experiences of bringing a case of homophobically motivated violence to CHRAJ, during which he was ignored and treated with disdain by CHRAJ staff. It also reflects an acute awareness of institutional homophobia and a deep-seated suspicion of national stakeholders involved in HIV and MSM health rights work. Community activists' suspicions tie into broader concerns over how development's prioritization of health has created financial incentives for government and civil society actors that are not supported by genuine commitment to MSM or LGBTI rights, as described in Chapter 2. As a result of this type of experience, a number of activists described their involvement in HIV initiatives as "tokenistic," especially since their voices are often ignored or marginalized within higher-level meetings or stakeholder events relating to HIV policy and prevention work. This dynamic again sheds light into the uneasy character of these alliances—the coalition of public health, government, NGO, and activist actors. It also suggest that the "carrot and stick" approach to tackling HIV and other sexual health rights in contexts where homosexuality is criminalized, that is, the attempt to incentivize otherwise hostile governments through aid funding and to put pressure on them through aid conditionality—leaves institutionalized homophobia largely intact (as well as intensifying political power struggles over sovereignty, as discussed Chapter 1).

Despite his experiences with institutions like CHRAJ, Francis avowed that he and his colleagues will not stop taking cases to the police, a commitment that is captured in his comment "But we help ourselves." Francis articulates a sense of self-determination that speaks to both his vision of community and collectivity and to his frustration with top-down, NGO-led interventions. These interventions are, according to Francis, not just inadequate or misguided, but shaped by false motives and opportunism. This, in turn, leaves queer working-class communities to "help themselves." Francis's emphasis on self-help and self-determination captures something of his spirit of defiance, his radicalism, and his commitment to fighting for justice, despite the myriad risks and challenges this entails.

CONCLUSION

While the practices and activities of queer community networks in Accra may not ostensibly be read as "activism," it is in these everyday acts of resistance that working-class queer individuals come together to challenge injustice, assert their rights, and unsettle heteronormativity, beyond the purview of NGO-led HIV and sexual rights work. As this chapter has shown, queer kinship arrangements, conflict mediation strategies, and practices of spatial queering are political in character and serve important material and affective functions for queer working-class Ghanaians. Furthermore, community activists' attempts to claim rights using existing legal mechanisms directly confront some of the primary political and institutional apparatus of homophobia in Ghana: the police and the legal system. In a context of entrenched heteronormativity and politicized homophobia, these are arguably some of the most subversive and dangerous political acts of all.

The four priorities for queer struggle examined in this chapter do not form part of a coherent manifesto or agreed set of aims and, compared to the fullest possible elaborations of LGBTI rights, might appear modest, fragmentary, or even unambitious in character. Similar priorities and rights (and indeed many others) are set out in the Yogyakarta Principles, for example, which were strategically—and, it has been suggested, conservatively—framed to reflect already recognized, as opposed to new, rights (Thoreson 2009).[11] Human rights scholars might also question whether, without decriminalization and the establishment of the fundamental rights of recognition and equality before the law, it is possible to address poverty, raise living standards, and improve employment opportunities for queer individuals in practice. These are, of course, valid practical and strategic concerns. Yet there is a sense in which this misses the underlying point. When Ghanaian activists say they want to realize rights for everybody, or that their struggle is equally about economic security, they are effectively rejecting the idea of autonomous struggle and highlighting the interconnectedness of different forms of injustice. In other words, they are tying LGBTI rights to a much broader desire for social, political, and economic change.

This is not meant to imply that Ghanaian community activists are expressly anticapitalist in their politics, although they are deeply opposed to inequality, injustice, and maldistribution. It is to recognize that meaningfully addressing these issues will require radical transformations in the political economy of development, in national legal systems and norms, and in relations of class, gender, race, and geopolitical power. To this end, the four priorities for queer struggle articulated by community activists (and embodied in their everyday practices of resistance) are not modest at all. Rather, they are crucial to understanding the character of queer oppression and resistance in Ghana, as well as the future possibilities of queer activism. They are also instructive for global actors—whether donor governments or activist groups based in the Global North—seeking to advance LGBTI rights in Ghana and other parts of Africa. At the very least, these actors must seek to better understand and work in solidarity with activists on the ground, in line with the strategies and priorities they identify for activism. This means looking beyond mainstream civil society organizations and beyond the remit of public health toward the practices of resistance that take place in the everyday.

Conclusion

The Current and Future Frontiers
of Queer African Activism

Because Africa is moving in several directions at once, this is a period that, at the same
time, has been, is not yet, is no longer, is becoming—in a state of preliminary outline
and possibility. The mirror reflects a figure that is in the present yet escapes it, that is, at
once, in front and behind, inside and outside, above and below, in the depths, and that is
hard to nail down.
   —Achille Mbembe, *On the Postcolony* (2001:241)

Africa must think beyond de-construction; after all, the term itself forces us back, time
and again, into the arms of the "colonial." So, ultimately, for Africans, the agenda for
decolonization and decolonial activism must involve *re*-constructions.
   —Sylvia Tamale, *Decolonization and Afro-feminism* (2020:21)

2019 was a year of both progress and setback for queer activists in Africa.
Legal battles in Botswana and Kenya over the status of domestic "against the
order of nature" laws highlight the multi-sited character of queer struggle
in the contemporary juncture, as well as the divergent paths being taken on
decriminalization in different country settings. This chapter surveys some
of these struggles and the strategies that underpin them. My intention is
not to impute a gradual or linear progression toward decriminalization
and the institution of formal LGBTI rights in Africa or, indeed, "to end off
[my] writing with a futuristic tone," as Matebeni's parodic essay suggests
(2014a:59). Rather, the chapter seeks to highlight the key part played by
activists in putting LGBTI rights and queer struggle on the political agenda,
the patchy and uneven distribution of prohibitions and protections across
different African settings, and the extent to which this landscape is subject to contestation and change. The second half of the chapter reads the

vision for queer liberation set out in the 2010 African LGBTI manifesto alongside the political priorities of queer community activists in Ghana, and contrasts this with the trajectories of mainstream queer activism in the Global North. In so doing, the chapter recaps the central arguments of this book: in essence, that political economy matters for queer struggle and, *vice versa*, that queer struggle matters for political economy. The chapter concludes that the liberatory potential of queer activism depends, in part, on some key political choices: between liberalism and radicalism, representation and redistribution, assimilation and transformation. Yet it will also be determined by our collective ability to forge transnational solidarities and to advance a queer-feminist, decolonial, and anti-capitalist political project for "the 99 per cent" (Arruzza et al. 2019).

THE CURRENT FRONTIERS OF STRUGGLE

Scholars have rightly drawn attention to the impact of colonial legacies and postcolonial power struggles in shaping the legal and political terrain of queer sexualities in Africa, including the rise of politicized homophobia and trends of expanded criminalization (Han and Mahoney 2018; Jjuuko and Tabengwa 2018; da Costa Santos and Waites 2019; see also Chapter 1). However, it is equally important to spotlight the role of queer and other African human rights organizations, activists, and community groups in forging resistance and affecting change, *and* in engendering pushbacks, big and small. Given how homosexuality has become bound up in questions of sovereignty, nationalism, identity, and culture in countries like Ghana—and the extent to which sexuality is an increasingly important locus of global governance and regulation—these pushbacks are almost inevitable; they occur whenever an oppressed, exploited, or otherwise minoritized group seeks to challenge injustice and inequality. Foregrounding this activism is also important in light of the narratives of "African homophobia" that circulate in some Western media discourse, which elide the diverse political activities of queer activists, organizations, community groups, and individuals taking place across the continent.

In the East African state of Kenya, activists have been organizing around the issue of decriminalization for a number of years, with the goal of repealing the country's penal code. Like Ghana's law, the Kenyan penal code dates back to the period of British colonial rule and criminalizes "carnal knowledge against the order of nature," which can result in up to fourteen years in prison, and "indecent practices between males," which can result in up to five years in prison.[1] In 2016, the National Gay and Lesbian Human Rights Commission, led by Eric Gitari, filed a petition challenging the country's "against the order of nature" laws. The petition argued that the laws on homosexuality stand in contradiction to the Kenyan constitution (an amended and updated version of which was promulgated in 2010). Referring to the provisions of the articles, Gitari's petition stated: "Those laws degrade the inherent dignity of affected individuals by outlawing their most private and intimate means of self-expression" (*Gitari v. Attorney General and another* 2016). The High Court of Kenya subsequently consolidated Gitari's submission with the Mathenge petition, put together by the Gay and Lesbian Coalition of Kenya and a number of other petitioners, which made similar claims regarding the unconstitutionality of the penal code in relation to the rights of equality, dignity, and privacy (Human Rights Watch 2019). The Mathenge petition went further to argue that the law goes against the provisions of the United Nations Universal Declaration of Human Rights and the African Charter on Human and Peoples Rights (*Mathenge and 7 others v. Attorney General* 2016).

In May 2019, a panel of three judges heard the case in the Kenyan High Court. They unanimously rejected the consolidated petition, stating: "We find that the impugned sections are not unconstitutional. Accordingly, the consolidated Petitions have no merit. We hereby decline the reliefs sought and dismiss the consolidated Petitions" (*Gitari and 7 others v. Attorney General* 2016). The judgment explained: "Looking at the impugned provisions *vis a vis* Article 45(2), we are satisfied that the provisions do not offend the right to privacy and dignity espoused in Articles 28 and 31 of the Constitution." While the decision came as a blow to activists in the country, they have since begun a process of appeal (Human Rights Watch 2023).

Just one month later, in June 2019, in the southern African country of Botswana, a similar case was being heard in the High Court in Gaberone. The petition in this instance was brought by an individual, Letsweletse Motshidiemang, with the Botswanan LGBTI organization LeGaBiBo supporting the case as amicus curiae (friend of the court).[2] The petition argued that Sections 164(a) and 167 of the Botswanan penal code—relating to "carnal knowledge of any person against the order of nature" and acts of "gross indecency with another person" respectively—were unconstitutional and violated the rights of liberty and privacy (*Motshidiemang v. Attorney General* 2019). In a landmark ruling, the three-judge panel unanimously agreed that sections of the

Botswana penal code were "unconstitutional." In particular, the judgment upheld the petition's argument that the law was incompatible with the right to privacy, with Judge Michael Leburu stating: "We have determined that it is not the business of the law to regulate private consensual sexual encounters." He added: "The state cannot be sheriff in people's bedrooms" (Brown 2019). Unlike in the Kenyan case, the Botswanan judgement explicitly framed the laws criminalizing homosexuality as a colonial inheritance and rejected the idea that homosexuality does not exist in Africa: "Sexual orientation is innate to human beings and is not a fashion statement. . . . Homosexuality is not un-African, but it is one other way Africans identify." The ruling continued, "Sodomy laws deserve a place in the museum or archives and not in the world" (Cotterill and Pilling 2019).

The Kenyan and Botswanan cases attracted considerable attention in national and transnational news media. Yet they are also the culmination of a series of smaller and less high-profile battles.[3] As such, their divergent outcomes are reflective of both country- and region-specific dynamics in the status and politicization of LGBTI rights. Since 2010, a number of African countries have repealed or removed laws that criminalize homosexuality: in January 2019, Angola amended its penal code to remove a "vices against nature" clause and to offer protection from discrimination on the grounds of sexual orientation; Lesotho decriminalized homosexual relations in 2010, followed by São Tome and Principe and Mozambique in 2014, and the Seychelles in 2016 (Mendos 2019). This means that all former Portuguese colonies in Africa have now decriminalized homosexuality. To put this into an even longer periodization, between 1969 and 2018 the percentage of UN member states in Africa that criminalize homosexuality fell by one-quarter, to 33 percent (Yang 2019:178).

The laws governing sexual orientation and gender identity across the African continent are evidently shifting and heterogeneous. However, the Kenyan and Botswanan legal cases also indicate that decriminalization—and more broadly the state—remains a key site of struggle when it comes to queer sexualities. As explored in the Ghanaian context in the introduction and Chapter 1, the state can play a key role in enabling or spearheading violence against queer communities, for example, by promoting anti-gay rhetoric, mobilizing politicized homophobia, and/or attempting to strengthen existing anti-homosexuality laws. Adrian Jjuuko and Monica Tabengwa describe this trend as "expanded criminalization," that is, "the process of building on existing laws to further criminalize same-sex conduct by adding to or reinterpreting them" (2018:64). One recent example of this is Ghana's proposed anti-LGBTQ+ bill, which is, at the time of writing, being debated in the Ghanaian parliament. Other examples include the ban placed on homosexual marriage by the Ugandan government in 2005, an act of expanded criminalization that was subsequently reproduced in Nigeria, Zimbabwe, Rwanda, the Democratic Republic of Congo, Liberia, Cameroon, Malawi, Kenya, Tanzania, and the Gambia (Jijuuko and Tabengwa 2018:63), and changes made by the Malawian government to the country's penal code in 2010, which outlawed consensual homosexual relations between women for the first time, with a punishment of up to five years in prison (Dunne 2012).

Rao (2014:171) argues that focusing on the legal norms and provisions governing sexual orientation and gender identity in Africa risks a form of state-centrism that obscures the realities of queer lived experience. Through mapping exercises such as the International Lesbian and Gay Association's State-Sponsored Homophobia report, Africa is invoked as a "spatial imaginary" where queer individuals are persecuted, imprisoned, and otherwise oppressed (in contrast to the "queer-friendly" state laws of the West). According to S.N. Nyeck (2021:2), this state-centrism relies on Western liberal ideas about modernity and "corporatist views about human rights, gender, and sexual identities," which are reflected in the activities of African LGBTI NGOs.

South Africa is a frequently cited example of the disconnect between state laws and queer lived experience, wherein comprehensive legal rights and protections for LGBTI individuals continue to be accompanied by high levels of homophobic and transphobic violence (Rao 2014; see also Ward 2013). On the other end of the spectrum—in legal terms at least—is Mauritania, where, as Epprecht (2013:3) highlights, US State Department investigations found no evidence of systematic oppression on the grounds of sexual orientation, despite one of the most draconian anti-homosexuality laws on the continent. Epprecht concludes that an ostensibly hostile legal environment may not always be mirrored in queer individuals' experiences of oppression. This builds on findings from other African contexts indicating that a lack of explicit vocabulary around queer sexual practices or identities does not necessarily correlate to forms of social stigma and discrimination (Tamale 2011; Morgan and Wieringa 2004; Epprecht 2008).

While I am sympathetic to these critiques of state-centrism and calls for greater nuance in understanding lived experience, the case of a queer Mauritanian man, "Ahmed A.," who was granted asylum in the United States in 2011, complicates some of Epprecht's claims. According to Ahmed's legal

team, "One of the difficulties in confronting Mauritania's violently homophobic law is that reported instances of state or tribal execution are not published. The Mauritanian government and the country's powerful tribal system often cover up their execution of LGBT individuals, recording other
causes of death" (Tran 2011). In this instance, a lack of evidence (or a culture
of silence around homosexuality) should not be conflated with less oppressive or violent experiences for queer individuals. Reflecting on West Africa,
activists and writers Ababacar Sadikh Ndoye and Emma Onekekou (2019)
similarly highlight how a sense of "false calm" and "deceptive silence" belies
the widespread violence and discrimination experienced by queer populations across the region. They further note that even in countries where there
is no law explicitly criminalizing homosexual relations, such as Côte d'Ivoire
and Burkina Faso, there are numerous documented cases of queer people
being targeted, prosecuted, imprisoned, and extorted by the police.

These complex dynamics suggest that decriminalization is not a pana-
cea for queer oppression, nor an end goal for queer struggle in itself. They
also underscore why fine-grained empirical research on queer sexualities is
needed, as a means to unsettle the West's cartographic imaginaries of sexual
modernization and to illuminate the varying contours of queer oppression
across different African settings. I would therefore agree that approaches to
struggle centered primarily or exclusively on the state may neglect other key
non-state sites of social and cultural power (Nyeck 2021), gloss the transnational ways in which homophobia is produced, both historically and contemporarily (Rao 2014; 2020), and work to reify and stabilize the state as site of
(sexual) governance (Puri 2016). At the same time, the experiences of activists in countries like Ghana, Kenya, and Botswana suggest that decriminalization does mark an important, if circumscribed, step toward the realization of
sexual justice. As the head of Botswana's LeGaBiBo, Anna Mmolai-Chalmers,
commented, following the decriminalization ruling in 2019: "We won't fool
ourselves. We know a change of law doesn't mean the end of discrimination.
But the law also has power" (Brown 2019).

In Ghana, recognition of the power of the law is even reflected in the testimony of some senior police personnel, namely Jones Blantari, the assistant
commissioner of police. During his time overseeing the Ghana Police Service's AIDS Control Program, Blantari became positioned as one of the more
"progressive" figures in the force on matters relating to sexuality. Blantari was
also involved in the values clarification work on sexual orientation and gender
identity organized by LGBTI/HIV NGOs in 2016. In an interview with Human

Rights Watch, Blantari stated clearly that the Ghanaian law was being used in repressive and punitive ways: "The term unnatural carnal knowledge is vague, does not have any clear meaning in law, creates difficulties in consistent interpretation and *its application is used to target LGBTI people*" (Human Rights Watch 2018:22, italics mine).[4] As the testimonies of CEPEHRG staff and other activists have demonstrated, without the fundamental right of equality before the law—and with a repressive penal code on the statute books—queer Ghanaians are extremely vulnerable to violence and discrimination, and encounter significant constraints on their ability to contest sexual and other forms of injustice. When viewed in strategic terms, the Ghanaian criminal code therefore represents a significant barrier to realizing the priorities for struggle identified by queer community activists: ending homophobic violence, addressing poverty, finding decent work, and improving mental health and well-being. In this sense, the horizon for queer struggle extends within and beyond the nation-state and its legal and regulatory apparatus.

Against this background, it may seem surprising that decriminalization and repeal of the unnatural carnal knowledge law have not historically been a key priority for Ghana's formal LGBTI/HIV organizations, as discussed in Chapter 3. The dominance of the sexual health agenda in global development goes some way to explain formal organizations' reticence on the issue of decriminalization. As described in Chapters 2 and 3, this overwhelming policy and programmatic focus has increasingly led groups like CEPEHRG away from more explicit LGBTI rights organizing toward sexual health advocacy on HIV, as part of a broader process of NGO-ization. This means that Ghanaian LGBTI/HIV organizations have largely avoided the state-centrism that has characterized some NGO-led activism on LGBTI rights in other parts of the continent (Nyeck 2021). But the case of CEPEHRG also demonstrates how this trajectory has been shaped and reinforced by a climate of politicized homophobia in Ghana, in which activists face serious threats to their safety. This shows how more "neutral" approaches to sexual rights in development can have both broadly *politicizing* effects, in the sense that they reiterate pathological accounts of queer sexuality and fuel moral panics, and specifically *depoliticizing* ones, in the sense that they encourage NGO-ization, draw activists away from more grassroots forms of organizing and reproduce class relations. As explored in Chapter 4, the proliferation of HIV prevention discourse centered on individualized notions of "behavior change" has also engendered complex ideational responses among queer men struggling to come to terms with their sexual orientation, namely by reinforcing internalized homophobia and cis-normativity.

On the issue of decriminalization, members of the Coalition Against Homophobia in Ghana (CAHG), a small umbrella group made up of various Ghanaian LGBTI/HIV and human rights NGOs, discussed the possibility of bringing a legal case for decriminalization in 2015, based on the incompatibility of the law with the Ghanaian constitution. Similar to the approach adopted by Botswanan and Kenyan activists, the case for incompatibility, it was suggested, could be made using the constitutionally enshrined right to privacy (or through an expanded interpretation of the constitutionally protected characteristic of sex). However, CAHG's discussions were sidelined in light of the deeply hostile atmosphere surrounding homosexuality in the public sphere at the time. In this sense, only time will tell if, when, and how Ghanaian activists seek to push for a repeal of the country's unnatural carnal knowledge law.

FROM SEXUAL HEALTH RIGHTS TO QUEER LIBERATION

The African LGBTI manifesto, written by a small group of activists at a roundtable event in Kenya in 2010, offers an expansive and all-encompassing view of queer liberation on the African continent. It is a statement that embeds queer liberation within a pan-Africanist vision of multidimensional struggle: against sexism, racism, material and spatial inequalities, violence, imperialism, neocolonialism, and environmental degradation:

> We stand for an African revolution which encompasses the demand for a re-imagination of our lives outside neo-colonial categories of identity and power. For centuries, we have faced control through structures, systems and individuals who disappear our existence as people with agency, courage, creativity, and economic and political authority.
>
> As Africans, we stand for the celebration of our complexities and we are committed to ways of being which allow for self-determination at all levels of our sexual, social, political and economic lives. The possibilities are endless. We need economic justice; we need to claim and redistribute power; we need to eradicate violence; we need to redistribute land; we need gender justice; we need environmental justice; we need erotic justice; we need racial and ethnic justice; we need

rightful access to affirming and responsive institutions, services and spaces; overall we need total liberation. (African LGBTI Manifesto 2010)[5]

I have included this extended excerpt in order to capture the spirit of the
statement and because it distills, in a sense, one of the central arguments
of this book: about the irreducibility and multiplicity of queer struggle.
The manifesto's vision of "total liberation" has far-reaching ramifications
for queer individuals and communities living across the African continent
and for the future trajectories—the "endless possibilities"—of queer African
activism. It also holds important insights for global development actors—
donor governments, international organizations, development agencies, and
NGOs—seeking to promote and support LGBTI rights. I read the theoretical
and strategic implications of this manifesto in conversation with the political
practices and priorities of queer activists in Ghana in the final section of this
chapter.

First, let me elaborate on the concept of queer liberation and what it
means in the context of this book. My usage of "queer liberation" is informed,
in part, by texts like the African LGBTI manifesto, as well as the case study
material and narrative testimonies of queer Ghanaians collected as part of
this research. It is intended to denote the difference between activism that
aims at (liberal) goals of "equality" and "empowerment"—which may center
on formal rights such as marriage, or as is more salient to the Ghanaian context, an instrumentalist form of "empowerment" intended to prevent disease
or reduce poverty—and activism that prioritizes (radical) goals of freedom,
justice, and redistribution, beyond the status quo. As this book has sought to
show, it is only by centring political economy that we we can fully understand
the roots and drivers of queer oppression in Ghana and why the struggle for
erotic justice is always also economic in character.

To help advance this argument, the book examined what the political
economy of development means in practice for the first wave of queer activist groups that emerged in Ghana during the late 1990s: the power relations
that determine the terms and conditions of their engagement in sexual health
and LGBTI rights work and how neoliberal economic rationalities shape the
terrain of NGO-led activism. In circumstances of scarce resources and politicized homophobia, one outcome is the adoption of corporate, professionalized NGO structures and funding models, which include top-down, technocratic, and managerialist practices that disconnect LGBTI/HIV NGOs from
the communities they are supposed to represent. Another outcome is the

take-up of peer education approaches to HIV prevention, as operationalized through development's neoliberal empowerment paradigm. This approach relies on and exploits the unpaid, caring labor of queer working-class men. In the Ghanaian context of widespread precarity, informality, and material hardship, this reinforces the co-constitutive effects of class and sexuality and places a disproportionate burden of responsibility on queer working-class men in tackling the HIV epidemic.

Against this background, Chapters 3 and 4 examined the lived experience of queer Ghanaian activists in order to shed light on the corporeality of development work on HIV, as well as the corporeality of activism. This analysis underscored the emotional and physical toll of queer organizing in the face of politicized homophobia and how activists navigate between structure and agency. As we saw in Adam Amoah's story, the structural violence of HIV is simultaneously lived as the structural violence of discrimination, homelessness, familial rejection, poverty, and isolation. Yet, Adam has "some spirit inside" him, a force that pushes him forward in his community activism, even when it is "too heavy" for him to carry.

Questions of embodiment are important for political economy because bodies are shaped by political, economic, and social forces; they are "deeply implicated in the reproduction of unequal power relations and, consequently, in questions of economic and social justice" (Smith 2018:108).[6] I would add that bodies are also deeply implicated in the daily acts of resistance that challenge injustice. In this sense, Adam's experiences demonstrate why sexual health approaches in development are failing to meet the needs and concerns of working-class queer communities, which go far beyond access to formal healthcare. These priorities were explored in detail in Chapter 4, which set out the everyday practices of resistance that characterize queer community networks in Accra, beyond the purview of development interventions on HIV and sexual health rights.

There are of course other important issues that arise from sexual health rights approaches in development that I have not addressed in depth in this book: the exclusion of women and of gender-nonconforming, transgender, and intersex individuals is one of the most important. While sexual rights approaches have proliferated in development discourse since the early 2000s, their orientation toward HIV prevention work means that, in practice, they have almost exclusively focused on men. In this sense, they represent another barrier to the advancement of queer struggle in the African context. This is true numerically in Ghana, since queer activism is constrained by the relatively small number of individuals who are actively and/or publicly involved, as well as strategically, since the struggle against homophobia and heteronormativity will not be successful without advances being made in other interrelated struggles: against patriarchy, sexism, racism, and class inequality. "Inter-movement solidarity," to borrow Currier's (2016) phrase, is therefore important in preventing queer activists and organizations from becoming too isolated (and vulnerable to repression and persecution), and in offering material and nonmaterial support, such as funding or support of a wider network of activists and supporters. While Currier conceptualizes grassroots organizations' links with foreign donors as "vertical solidarity partnerships" (2016:147), the Ghanaian case suggests this is, at best, an optimistic way of framing it. These "partnerships" are in reality highly unequal, particularly given the geopolitics of foreign aid, the power asymmetries between donors and implementing partners (both internationally and nationally), and their transformative and, at times, divisive effects on existing queer formations.[7]

WHY QUEER STRUGGLE MATTERS FOR POLITICAL ECONOMY

Reflecting on the field of Marxist theory in 2006, Marxist feminist scholar Rosemary Hennessy argued that "those who are thinking critically about sexuality are few and far between" (2006:388). It is not altogether surprising, therefore, that queer theory—an entire field of scholarship dedicated to the study and interrogation of sexuality—has had an uneasy, if not altogether fractious, relationship with Marxism (Ferguson 2004; Binnie 2004; Lewis 2016; see also Smith 2016). In theoretical terms, this is typically attributed to disagreements over the primacy of the "cultural" or the "economic" and to perceived inadequacies in orthodox Marxist theorizing on gender, sexuality, and race. In the field of political economy, the most frequently referenced example of these tensions is the debate between Nancy Fraser and Judith Butler, prompted by the publication of Fraser's 1997 book, *Justice Interruptus*. In this work, Fraser sets out a critical theoretical framework that distinguishes between "injustices of distribution" and "injustices of recognition," in order to understand the rise of the New Left in Europe and North America post-1945. Gay and lesbian movements, in Fraser's terminology, essentially entail struggles over recognition, while working-class movements entail struggles over distribution. Butler addressed this typology in their provocatively entitled piece "Merely Cultural," which challenged orthodox Marxist reactions to the "cultural turn" and a secondary, related tendency to dis-embed queer struggle from political economy. They argue: "Whereas class and race struggles are understood as pervasively economic and feminist struggles to be sometimes economic and sometimes cultural, queer struggles are understood not only to be cultural struggles, but to typify the 'merely cultural' form that contemporary social movements have assumed" (Butler 1998:38).

I agree that Fraser's framework unhelpfully reifies a culture/economy, social life / material life binary, in which sexual injustices are seen as somehow epiphenomenal to the economic. However, there is also a sense in which the protagonists of this debate are talking at cross-purposes, since Fraser is making a theoretical rather than ontological distinction between these two types of injustice in the context of a "postsocialist" decoupling of identity-based struggles from class-based ones. Moreover, she clearly distances herself, as Butler acknowledges, from the economistic strands of Marxism toward which Butler directs critique. The Fraser-Butler debate remains valuable, nonetheless, in that it brings to the fore fundamental questions about the relationship between sexuality, class, culture, and economy, as well as the implications of "identity politics" for queer activism in different parts of the world.[8] In the context of queer oppression and struggle in Ghana, the attempt to disentangle injustices of recognition from injustices of redistribution is all but impossible at the level of people's everyday everyday lives.

What I have tried to draw out in this book, in fact, is the extent to which queer Ghanaian's experiences of sexual oppression and injustice *cannot* be separated from their experiences of economic inequality and exploitation (and how these relations are simultaneously racialized, gendered, and territorialized). This is not to suggest that these injustices are the same thing in a phenomenological sense, but that this creates a powerful nexus of oppression that is both cultural and economic in character. To impose a chronology on these injuries—that is, the idea that the (economic) maldistribution arises from the (cultural) misrecognition—is rather a chicken-and-egg exercise that obscures more than it illuminates. It also misses a more fundamental point about how sexual injustices are constitutive of—that is, rather than incidental to, or external from—the global capitalist economy. As set out in detail in Chapter 1, structures of racialized heteronormativity have material and cultural bases, which encompass the gender division of labor, family and household arrangements, and relations of production and reproduction, as well as being structured by state and supra-state modes of governance. This means that it is empirically and theoretically unsustainable to dichotomize

queer sexuality and economy; the logics of hetero- and homonormativity—
the complex web of social relations that normalize and naturalize sexual and
gender difference—cannot be unraveled from the logics of global capitalism.
Nor can they be disentangled from the afterlives of colonialism.

Addressing the issue of criminalization—ostensibly an "injustice of
recognition"—would evidently not address the vast socioeconomic inequalities that shape working-class queer life in Ghana. At the same time, it is
difficult—but not impossible, as the attempts of some Ghanaian activists
illustrate—to tackle other inequalities without simultaneously remedying
this lack of recognition. As Fraser herself acknowledges, "In the real world,
of course, culture and political economy are always imbricated with one
another; and *virtually every struggle against injustice, when properly understood, implies demands for both redistribution and recognition*" (1997:12, italics
mine). In this sense, I return to the recognition versus redistribution debate
for practical as well as theoretical reasons: because it has implications for how
queer activists conceptualize the issues on which they organize and the overarching frameworks they use to guide them. However, this categorical separation is frequently not the way in which injustice is experienced, embodied,
and resisted at the microlevel of queer lives.

While the precise relationship between sexuality, hetero- and homonormativity, and capitalism is likely to remain the subject of debate, queer theory's push to uncouple and deconstruct naturalized sex and gender norms is
evidently far from incompatible with the core concerns of political economy.
Indeed, expanding our ambit from Marxist feminist scholarship to include
the diversity of feminist political economy, it becomes clear that questions of
gender, sexuality, and body politics have long been centralized. The project
of feminist political economy has thus entailed interrogating how "gender
operates as a relation of social power" (Elias and Roberts 2018: 4) in the global
economy and documenting the drivers of gender oppression and inequality—as these play out and are reproduced across multiple scales of governance
and spheres of power. This book has sought to move this project forward by
examining the materiality of queer oppression and resistance in Ghana, using
a queer political economy approach. I premised this approach on three key
assumptions:

1. Sexuality, like gender, is a legitimate and important topic of academic inquiry in political economy, and, similarly, studies of African
   sexualities can be enriched by integrating a queer political economy
   perspective;

2. We cannot understand the impact of global development agendas focused on sexual rights without interrogating their imbrication in hetero- and homonormative structures, institutions, and governance regimes; processes of capitalist restructuring; historical and ongoing forms of (colonial-)capitalist accumulation and dispossession; and queer people's everyday intimate and affective lives, including relations of (re)production;

3. The injuries that arise from sexual orientation and/or gender identity are not just incidental to, or even intensified by, broader inequalities and hierarchies within the global economy, but are (re)productive of it.

I operationalized my queer political economy approach using three core dimensions for analysis: sexuality, capitalism, and the state; sexuality, capitalism, and global governance; and the everyday political economies of queer oppression and resistance. Queer political economy is, in this sense, not only useful for understanding the character of activism in Ghana—and the ways in which global development processes shape and reconfigure this landscape— but offers a powerful lens for examining and highlighting the relationship between different struggles across space and time.

WHY POLITICAL ECONOMY MATTERS FOR QUEER STRUGGLE

In the Global North, a tug-of-war is taking place over the heart and soul of queer politics. Writing this chapter in the month of June, now known as "Pride month" in much of Europe and North America, I am struck by the sheer ubiquity of the rainbow flag. Once a symbol of struggle for the gay and lesbian movement, the flag can now be found adorning everything from banks to buses, supermarkets to sandwiches. Walking through the Soho district of Central London recently, I mistook an outlet of the Wagamama's restaurant chain for a gay bar. Seeking to capitalize on Pride month celebrations, the restaurant had adopted the colors and stripes of the rainbow flag to appeal to (and confuse) the district's passing crowds. The commodification and corporatization of queer struggle is especially striking in formerly queer but now hypergentrified London neighborhoods like Soho. The rainbow flag, in this new order of things, is a central part of the iconography of pink capitalism.

There is an established literature—across media, activist, and academic spheres—critiquing the co-optation of queer liberation by forms of state and corporate pinkwashing (Schulman 2011), complexes of homonationalism

(Puar 2007), and the growing influence of a new queer politics shaped by neoliberalism (Hennessy 2000; Duggan 2002; Binnie 2004; Cohen 2005; Altman 2012). Lisa Duggan (2002:190) has dubbed this political shift the "New Homonormativity," in which key tenets of gay politics are reinscribed. She argues that "'equality' becomes narrow, formal access to a few conservatizing institutions, 'freedom' becomes impunity for bigotry and vast inequalities in commercial life and civil society, the 'right to privacy' becomes domestic confinement, and democratic politics itself becomes something to be escaped." In other words, since the 1990s, a dominant model of queer politics has prioritized representation and recognition over more structural, redistributive demands, as part of a trend toward autonomous, "single issue" struggle, to borrow Audre Lorde's (2007:138) phrase, and a broader privatization of sexuality (Floyd 2009).

As the Black feminist scholar and activist Barbara Smith commented in 2019: "We have won rights and achieved recognition that would have been unimaginable 50 years ago, but many of us continue to be marginalized, both in the larger society and within the movement itself." In this way, the new homonormativity works to conceal the connections between LGBTI rights, queer oppression, and other key social and economic justice issues, including anti-racist and anti-capitalist politics.

As this discussion suggests, the battle over queer politics is, in part, a battle over what ideals, principles, and strategies should animate contemporary queer movements in countries like the United Kingdom and the United States (and what factors have led these social movements into the position they find themselves today). Duggan's analysis indicates that addressing the new homonormativity will require an interrogation of wider shifts in the political economy of sexual identities, activism, and citizenship under neoliberalism. In particular, this means reclaiming the "gay agenda" from a narrow focus on formal equality and legal rights—what Duggan and Kim (2012) call "marriage, military and markets" and a "trickle-down" approach to gay rights based on greater representation—to consider the issues that affect the 99 percent: "economic justice, housing, health care, welfare, immigration, sexual liberation, aging, disability, gender identity and expression, HIV/AIDS, rural and urban community organizing, public space, sex work, drugs, crime, policing and prisons, reproductive rights, racial injustice, and more." Put simply, northern LGBTI movements should move beyond "queer liberalism" (Eng 2010) and do more to prioritize matters of economic, gender, and racial justice. This is a call to recover the radical, redistributive traditions of queer struggle (and materialist modes of analysis) and to repurpose them for the contemporary juncture. As Barbara Smith (2019) emphasizes: "Unless we eradicate the systemic oppressions that undermine the lives of the majority of LGBTQ people, we will never achieve queer liberation."

An in-depth discussion of mainstream gay and lesbian activism in the Global North as it links to the sexual politics of neoliberalism is beyond the scope of this chapter. What I wish to focus on, however, are the implications of these experiences for other forms of queer struggle and movement building around the world. This is not a teleological, sexual modernization analysis, and I am not implying that countries like Ghana will, or should, follow similar paths toward the institutionalization of LGBTI rights and the proliferation of identity-based struggles (indeed there is already a vast literature on the complex and problematic impacts of "queer globalization," as discussed in Chapter 1). Duggan and Kim's primary reference point is the United States, where the political economic landscape of queer sexual citizenship and identity differs significantly from the landscape in Ghana. A critique of the prioritization of formal rights and recognition at the expense of more all-encompassing concerns may therefore seem decidedly disconnected from the struggles of working-class Ghanaians, some of which are, as this book has documented, about meeting basic needs. Yet the call to reorient and reclaim queer politics resonates with the African LGBTI manifesto—with its push to reimagine queer lives "outside neo-colonial categories of identity"— and, importantly, with the refusal to abstract queer struggle from other forms of economic and social justice among queer community activists in Ghana. The vision of struggle articulated by these activists is, in an important way, opposed to the kind of single-issue, identity-based struggles that have characterized mainstream queer/LGBTI movements in North America and Europe over the past three decades. It insists instead on the indivisibility of redistribution and recognition and on envisioning justice outside the narrow confines of (neoliberal) sexual citizenship.

Building on the earlier discussion of decriminalization, this understanding of struggle also helps to explain why the attainment of anti-discrimination laws or marriage rights does not equate to queer liberation, especially for poor and working-class queer people; queer people with insecure immigration status; and Black, indigenous, and queer people of color, irrespective of geography. In the aftermath of the 2008 global financial crisis, for example, homelessness, unemployment, and precarity rose sharply among LGBTI young people in the United States, particularly trans young people and young people of color (Duggan and Kim 2012). In the United Kingdom, LGBTI individuals have disproportionately borne the brunt of austerity, with especially disastrous consequences for their ability to access services, such as mental health support (see Smith 2018). While the effects of these interconnected phenomena—crisis and austerity—are mediated by differences of race, gender, class, age, and citizenship, the parallels with the stories of queer individuals in this book—of homelessness, unemployment, economic hardship, and poor mental health—are stark.

In Ghana, strategic dilemmas, debates, and disagreements over how to frame and organize around LGBTI rights and sexual injustice are only likely to proliferate, especially in the current context of politicization, which includes an expanding number of dedicated queer activist groups and organizations, as well as increasingly violent forms of state repression. If we take the experiences of mainstream LGBTI movements in the Global North seriously, the liberatory potential of this organizing depends, in part, on the outcome of these dilemmas, on how activists navigate between liberalism and radicalism, representation and redistribution, assimilation and transformation. At the same time, the strategic agency of this small group of actors should not be overstated, not least because, as this book has shown, their activities are delimited by vastly unequal power relations and forms of structural violence. This means that queer liberation in Ghana cannot be realized without forging connections across struggles and without building transnational solidarities. To this end, there is practical as well as empirical urgency in deconstructing a Global North / Global South binary when it comes to assessing the state of queer struggle, particularly since considerable transnational media concern over homophobia has converged around Africa. Not only does this reinforce colonial tropes of Africa as "backward" and "uncivilized," and ignore the ways in which queer Africans are coming together to contest heteronormativity, it takes attention away from the connections between different struggles and their transnational character: to paraphrase the African LGBTI manifesto, it disguises the intimate links between economic, gender, environmental, erotic, and racial injustices.

What I am arguing, therefore, and what I have sought to demonstrate in this book, is that these struggles are interconnected because they are fundamentally about political economy: that advancing or expanding queer individuals' knowledge of HIV or STIs, improving their access to and experiences of healthcare, and building their knowledge of sexual health issues is insufficient to address the materiality of homophobia and oppression. If we are to see meaningful progress toward rights, freedom, and justice within and *beyond* the status quo, we have to take into account the political economic systems, institutions, and norms that shape everyday queer life and the lives of other oppressed groups around the world. Theoretically, this means rejecting narrow epistemological, theoretical, or disciplinary lenses in the study of queer struggle and bringing into view a broad range of relations that encompass households, states, markets, international financial institutions, international organizations, and development agencies. It means considering sexual injustices in relation to trajectories of capitalist restructuring and crisis, and their entanglement in the afterlives of colonialism. Unsettling a Global North / Global South binary in the study of queer politics is again crucial here, because it illuminates why liberation is contingent on redressing global inequalities in the distribution of land, income, wealth, power, and capital that are historically embedded and contemporarily reproduced. This is the context in which Ghanaian activists locate their activism and speaks to what Angela Davis refers to as "not so much the intersectionality of identities, but the intersectionality of struggles" (2016:144). This argument also builds on long-standing work from scholars of African development that shows how the future of African liberation is entwined in domestic, continental, and global political economy (Nkrumah 1965; Amin 1971; Rodney 1972; Tamale 2020). As Tamale (2020:35) emphasizes, decolonial liberation requires the "dismantling of the neoliberal capitalist system."

LGBTI RIGHTS AND GLOBAL DEVELOPMENT

It would be remiss of me to write a book about queer activism in Ghana that highlights the limitations of sexual health rights agendas and frameworks in development without reflecting on alternative approaches and ways forward for global actors—donor governments, development agencies, international organizations, international NGOs, and activists groups—seeking to support and promote LGBTI rights globally and in Africa in particular. One hot topic within development circles has been the question of aid conditionality. While the literature on aid conditionality in general has mixed views on its purposes and effectiveness (see, for example, Mosley et al. 2004; Fisher 2015), the approach has continued to prove popular among European and North American donor governments. Following the passage of the Anti-Homosexuality Bill in Uganda in 2015, for example, the United States, the Netherlands, Denmark, Sweden, and Norway all withdrew or suspended elements of development funding from the Ugandan government (Carroll and Itaborahy 2015). However, aid conditionality, as a tool to promote and protect LGBTI rights, has been criticized by both scholars and activists alike (khanna 2011; Dunne 2012; Pambazuka 2011; Johnson 2011; Vrede 2020), including though a number of public statements. In 2011, for example, a coalition of African civil society groups, activists, and individuals came together to ask northern governments to stop using (or threatening) aid conditionality as a response to infringements on LGBTI rights. They stated:

> A vibrant social justice movement within African civil society is working to ensure the visibility of—and enjoyment of rights by—LGBTI people. . . . Donor sanctions are by their nature coercive and reinforce the disproportionate power dynamics between donor countries and recipients. They are often based on assumptions about African sexualities and the needs of African LGBTI people. They disregard the agency of African civil society movements and political leadership. They also tend, as has been evidenced in Malawi, to exacerbate the environment of intolerance in which political leadership scapegoat LGBTI people for donor sanctions in an attempt to retain and reinforce national state sovereignty. (Pambazuka 2011)

As this excerpt indicates, queer African activists and civil society organizations are critical of the unequal power dynamics that underpin donor threats to impose aid conditionalities and their wider disregard for the strategies and agency of queer African activists and communities. The point that sanctions are "often based on assumptions about African sexualities and the needs of African LGBTI people" highlights one key reason why exogenous, top-down interventions and "solutions" from donor governments are so unpopular. In Ghana, staff from CEPEHRG, a signatory of the 2011 statement, were strongly opposed to the linking of aid conditionalities to LGBTI rights. They released their own independent statement, through CAHG, stating that aids cuts "will rather stigmatize these groups and individuals. LGBTI people will be used as scapegoats for government inability to support its citizens" (Coalition against Homophobia in Ghana 2011).[9] Conditionalities are therefore seen as counterproductive, not just because of the risk of backlash and

scapegoating, but because queer communities are impacted, often disproportionately, by the human and economic development issues that foreign aid is
supposed to target.

The way to address these dynamics is at once simple and extraordinarily
complex. If readers take away only one thing from this book it should be
that external actors must listen to the diverse needs, views, and priorities
of queer African communities themselves. This may seem self-evident, but
the disregard with which donor governments, development agencies, and
other funders treat queer African activists is a consistent thread in public
statements, such as those released in 2011, and in the testimonies of Ghanaian activists. Where development actors do engage with and seek to support
the work of queer social movements in Africa, they must look outside formalized NGO spaces and connect with more grassroots networks of queer
(working-class) individuals. At the very least, this is vital in understanding
why particular development agendas and paradigms are not working and,
in some instances, are making things worse. Beyond that, the findings of
this book indicate that the task at hand is a much bigger and more far-
reaching one. It is a task that requires us to build alternatives to neoliberal
modes of global governance and development, to put an end to expropria-
tion and exploitation, and to dismantle the hierarchies of gender, race, sexuality, ability, citizenship, and geography upon which the global economy
rests. This project will be difficult but not insurmountable; as Harsha Walia
reminds us, "Injustice is not ordained to determine our future. Empires
crumble, capitalism is not inevitable, gender is not biology, whiteness is not
immutable, prisons are not inescapable, and borders are not natural law"
(2021:215).

A LUTA CONTINUA

For those of us invested in the struggle for queer liberation, the current moment could understandably fill us with despair. Against the backdrop of a
heterogeneous and increasingly global anti-gender movement, the rights of
queer and trans people across many parts of the world are under attack. In the
African context, progress in decriminalization and the institution of formal
LGBTI rights in some settings has paralleled retrenchment, repression, and
backlash elsewhere. The testimonies of queer Ghanaian men collected in this

book reveal the powerful intersections of race, class, sexuality, and geography and the myriad ways in which "*sasso* life is not easy." Yet these testimonies should also be a source of inspiration. In the face of politicized homophobia and profound structural inequalities, the transgressive power of queer Ghanaian activism—the quotidian acts of defiance and community, subversion and solidarity—and the moments where queer people "live like they want to live" are rendered even more poignant, even more arresting. This kind of activism reminds us of the potential for small acts, micropractices, and human hope itself to push the course of history in a different direction.

APPENDIX A

Discussed in the Prologue, the Gay and Lesbian Association of Ghana (GALAG) issued a statement in 2006 addressing media rumors about an "international gay conference" that was purportedly being held in Ghana. Their full statement appears here, as was made available by the International Gay and Lesbian Human Rights Commission.

GAY AND LESBIAN ASSOCIATION OF GHANA SPEAKS OUT ON RECENT ATTACKS

SEPTEMBER 15, 2006

The Gay and Lesbian Association of Ghana feels compelled to issue this statement in the face of mounting misinformation being made public in both print and electronic media about an alleged two-day international gay conference, supposedly coming on in Accra International Conference Centre and in Koforidua, respectively. We wish to clarify several issues here:

1. The Gay & Lesbian Association of Ghana (GALAG) has never discussed, nor have we ever organised, an international Lesbian/Gay/Bisexual/Transgender [LGBT] conference in Ghana. Since our Executive President appeared in some electronic media, this conference appears to have been the brainchild of someone's vivid imagination. As an association, we are not prepared to organise such a conference anywhere in Ghana, let alone any part of the universe, at this point.
2. We have no hand in—nor the faintest clue about—any such conference to be organised by any group anywhere; neither do we know of—nor

have we heard of—any such event. All we know is what is being ped-
dled irresponsibly in the media, apparently oblivious to the journalis-
tic ethical code which calls for confirming such a potentially controversial event with at least two or three reliable sources before putting it
on air or in print media as truth.

3. GALAG is like any other non-governmental association representing a
population which exercises its constitutional rights, votes in elections,
pays our taxes, cares for our parents, children, siblings and other family members, working dutifully at our jobs and, therefore, contributing
our fair share to national growth.

4. We wish to state categorically that GALAG does not promote homosexuality, but rather seeks the sexual well-being of same-gender-loving
people, their families and friends, as well as the general population at
large. LGBTI individuals and their loved ones are frequently rejected
and have no place to turn. GALAG tries to fill that void.

5. We work hard to promote the well-being and health of same-gender-
loving people trying to survive in an otherwise hostile environment.

6. We have no clear estimate of the number of GLBT in Ghana, but ini-
tial studies here have shown that about half of Ghanaian men who
have sex with other men are also having sex with women, creating a
potential "crossover" for HIV/STDs between the gay and heterosexual
populations here. As for sheer numbers, it is safe to say that about 10%
of the Ghanaian population—or approximately 2 million Ghanaians—
have been involved in same-sex sexual relationships. During the past
year, through brief research GALAG has participated in, nearly 2,000
of these have been identified in Accra and Tema alone. Each of these
men & women contributes positively to Ghanaian life.

7. We have peer educators who do outreach in the LGBTI community to
educate vulnerable community members on such issues as safer sexual
practices, accessing user-friendly health and social services, and generally to discuss their well-being. This is only necessary because many
of them cannot receive the nurturing they deserve from their families,
their churches, their mosques, their schools or other social institutions
which so readily provide needed support to heterosexual individuals.

8. Homosexuality has been with humans from the beginning of time.
Some of our brothers and sisters, daughters and sons, mothers and
fathers or other family members may be involved in same-gender-

loving and need the same support we would easily offer them if they were heterosexual. Those who would quote the Bible, the Koran, the Talmud or any other such religious document need only remember that all religions of the world have a variation on: "judge not, lest ye be judged." As for Leviticus and Corinthians, we need only look deeper to see that, as a culture, we are not willing to condone slavery, to stone women in red dresses, to reject men who shave their beards or people who eat shellfish, all of which are also in the Bible. So why should we single out this one population, LGBT, for our anger and hatred, based on scriptures? Hatred is not a good family value for our children to be taught.

9. Homosexuality touches every home, every work place, every church and every mosque in Ghana. We hope that all caring and intelligent Ghanaians would never be influenced or moved to hatred by lies from some unknown hate-mongering group or individuals trying to stir up controversy by fraudulently claiming to organize a gay conference in the name of this association.

10. Media personnel and the public need to be careful stereotyping homosexuality in the newspapers, on radio and TV. We have found lots of the comments and reactions to homosexuality to be weightless and prove the general public's ignorance of lesbian, gay, bisexual and transgendered individuals. We are everywhere—albeit many of us "closeted" because of anti-gay sentiment, harassment and violence, when we should instead be protected by the constitution to be able to achieve our potential, like any other Ghanaian should.

FOOD FOR THOUGHT

1. How many Ghanaian mothers and fathers will kill their sons or daughters for being gay?
2. How many elders in the church or mosque will lay down their church or mosque roles because they are "gay" or "bisexual"?
3. Let he or she who is without sin cast the first stone!! We know that God and Allah are for truth and compassion, while some men and women prefer to gossip, lie and breed hatred. We come out on the side of truth and compassion.

For further information, please feel free to contact us at either of the e-mail addresses below.

Prince Kweku MacDonald,
Gay & Lesbian Association of Ghana (GALAG)

Source: An archived source is available here: https://web.archive.org/ web/20061025182129/http://www.iglhrc.org/site/iglhrc/section.php?detail=679&id=5 (accessed January 10, 2022).

AFRICAN LGBTI MANIFESTO/DECLARATION

As discussed in the Conclusion, the African LGBTI manifesto was written by a small group of activists in Kenya in 2010. Their full manifesto appears here, courtesy of the African Activist Archive.

APRIL 18, 2010, NAIROBI, KENYA

As Africans, we all have infinite potential. We stand for an African revolution which encompasses the demand for a re-imagination of our lives outside neo-colonial categories of identity and power. For centuries, we have faced control through structures, systems and individuals who disappear our existence as people with agency, courage, creativity, and economic and political authority.

As Africans, we stand for the celebration of our complexities and we are committed to ways of being which allow for self-determination at all levels of our sexual, social, political and economic lives. The possibilities are endless. We need economic justice; we need to claim and redistribute power; we need to eradicate violence; we need to redistribute land; we need gender justice; we need environmental justice; we need erotic justice; we need racial and ethnic justice; we need rightful access to affirming and responsive institutions, services and spaces; overall we need total liberation.

We are specifically committed to the transformation of the politics of sexuality in our contexts. As long as African LGBTI people are oppressed, the whole of Africa is oppressed.

This vision demands that we commit ourselves to:

- Reclaiming and sharing our stories (past and present), our lived realities, our contributions to society and our hopes for the future;
- Strengthening ourselves and our organizations, deepening our links and understanding of our communities, building principled alliances, and actively contributing towards the revolution.
- Challenging all legal systems and practices which either currently criminalize or seek to reinforce the criminalization of LGBTI people, organizations, knowledge creation, sexual self expression, and movement building.
- Challenging state support for oppressive sexual, gendered, discriminatory norms, legal and political structures and cultural systems.
- Strengthening the bonds of respect, cooperation, passion, and solidarity between LGBTI people, in our complexities, differences and diverse contexts. This includes respecting and celebrating our multiple ways of being, self expression, and languages.
- Contributing to the social and political recognition that sexuality, pleasure, and the erotic are part of our common humanity.
- Placing ourselves proactively within all movement building supportive of our vision.

End!

Source: A PDF of the manifesto is available here: https://www.fahamu.org/mbbc/wp-content/uploads/2011/09/African-LGBTI-Manifesto-2010.pdf (accessed January 10, 2022).

APPENDIX C

As discussed in the Conclusion, the CAHG statement made in 2011 includes CEPEHRG, among other groups, as signatories. Their full press release appears here.

PRESS RELEASE ON THE BRITISH PRIME MINISTER'S "HOMOSEXUALITY THREAT" TO GHANA FROM THE COALITION AGAINST HOMOPHOBIA IN GHANA

ACCRA, 03 NOVEMBER, 2011

The Coalition against Homophobia in Ghana (CAHG), the Gay and Lesbian Association of Ghana (GALAG) and other LGBTI Networks in Ghana are surprised and in total shock at the increased interest by the UK government to withdraw aid to some African countries who are homophobic. Though the Coalition have no problem with calling on government to abide by the British code of conduct for financial support, we believe LGBTI people do not live in isolation in Africa. We have families and friends who need these aids to survive on daily basis.

Cutting aid to some selected Africa countries due to homophobic laws therefore will not help the LGBTI people in these countries, but will rather stigmatize these groups and individuals. LGBTI people will be used as scape goats for government inability to support its citizens and some sectors of the economy.

The challenge now is that:

1. Homosexuality is now being seen as western import due to the continuous threats from the UK government. It is now difficult to convince the ordinary person on the street that homosexuality was not imported into Africa; although we know and have always had African indigenous people who are born homosexuals.
2. LGBTI groups and organizations are finding it very difficult and risky to organize their programs due to such threats and continuous discussion on radio and television stations in Ghana.
3. Support from government agencies for LGBTI programs with regards to health will be affected since the government will not want to be seen as promoting or supporting LGBTI activities in the country. We believe the UK government can use diplomacy to get some of these important issues across to the countries noted for promoting hate against homosexuals or the LGBTI community in Africa. We encourage the UK government to find other alternative way to address the issue other than this option, which is going to increase the level of stigma, violence and discrimination against LGBTI people in Africa.

Though all these noise[s] continue to go against LGBTI groups and individuals in Africa, development partners never supports [*sic*] LGBTI initiatives on the ground. Embassies and consulates including the EU offices continue to turn deaf ears to LGBTI issues insisting that their priorities do not include LGBTI people in Africa.

We are by this release appealing to development partners to channel some support to LGBTI groups and organization in countries like Ghana to support local or internal advocacy as well as network building with state institutions.

This we believe will go a long way to help the LGBTI people in Ghana and Africa at large.

For more information, please contact the coalition on coalition.homophobia.gh@gmail.com

Signed:

1. Coalition against Homophobia in Ghana
2. Centre for Popular Education and Human Rights, Ghana
3. Gay and Lesbian Association of Ghana (GALAG)

4. Face AIDS Ghana
5. National Association of Persons Living with HIV/AIDS (NAP+)
6. Development Communication Initiatives—Ghana
7. Young People Advocate for a Change
8. Youth and Human Rights—Ghana

Source: The press release as posted on the African Activist Archive is available here: http://africanactivistarchive.blogspot.com/2011/11/lgbti-activists-say-no-to-uk-prime.html (accessed January 10, 2022).

NOTES

PROLOGUE

1. As Akua Gyamerah (2021:126) explains, not only did media reports on the Eastern Region "registrations" conflate homosexuality with HIV and sexually transmitted infections (STIs)—i.e., by implying that the majority of the eight thousand people had HIV or an STI—but cited incorrect figures regarding both estimated numbers of men who have sex with men in the region and HIV prevalence. This incident was particularly significant since it was one the first occasions when information (albeit misrepresented) from a donor-funded workshop on HIV/STI prevention was used by the Ghanaian media as the basis for claims about the growth of homosexuality (Gyamerah 2021).

2. In the interests of confidentiality and safety, all research participants have been given a pseudonym. The names of the LGBTI/HIV organizations and other NGOs who participated in this research have not been pseudonymized, with the consent of their executive directors.

3. For a detailed discussion of the "homoconference" controversy see Dankwa 2021.

4. The full GALAG statement is reproduced in Appendix A.

5. There is considerable variation, however, in the laws governing homosexuality across the African continent, including in West Africa (see Conclusion).

6. Some prominent (but far from exhaustive) examples include the photography of visual artist and activist Zunele Muholi, which depicts queer lives in South Africa; the NEST collective's *Stories of Our Lives* (2014), an anthology of short films exploring the real-life experiences of queer individuals in Kenya; and the writings of acclaimed Kenyan author Binyavanga Wainana, whose work includes the moving autobiographical piece "I Am a Homosexual, Mum," published in 2014. In the Ghanaian context, the photographer Eric Gyamfi's *Just Like Us* (2016) series documented the everyday lives of queer people in Ghana. The series was exhibited at Accra's Nubuke Foundation (for a discussion of its reception see Adjepong 2021).

7. According to Ann McClintock (1995:22), the genealogy of these ideas can be traced back through centuries of European writing about Africa and the Americas. She notes: "Long before the era of high Victorian imperialism, Africa and the Americas had become what can be called a porno-tropics for the European imagination—a fantastic

magic lantern of the mind onto which Europe projected its forbidden sexual desires and fears."

8. Achille Mbembe (2001:2) offers a compelling analysis of the discursive construction of African "otherness," which highlights how Africa "as an idea, a concept, has historically served, and continues to serve, as a polemical argument for the West's desperate desire to assert its difference from the rest of the world."

INTRODUCTION

1. This observation is not wholly new, since it is already acknowledged that, in practice, there is extensive overlap between rights-based and public health approaches (Epprecht 2013:149).

2. In May 2023 the International Monetary Fund (IMF) approved a loan of approximately $3 billion to support the Ghanaian government to deal with the crisis, as part of its "Post COVID-19 Program for Economic Growth" (IMF 2023).

3. *Trotro* refers to one of the privately owned minibuses that operate as a form of public transport throughout Ghana. *Trotro* is commonly believed to derive from the Ga word for three pence, *tro*, as during colonial times the cost of a ride was three pence (Okoye 2010).

4. *Kayayei* (sing. *kayaye*) can be translated as "women head-porters", from the Hausa *kaya*, "to carry," and the Ga *yei*, "women" (Opare 2003:34).

5. I am borrowing Saidiya Hartman's (2006) usage of "afterlife" here, in lieu of the more common term "legacies," to capture how the power relations of the colonial *durée* continue to "live on" and constitute the political economy of the postcolonial era. Writing on the United States, Hartman (2006:6) explains: "Black lives are still imperiled and devalued by a racial calculus and a political arithmetic that were entrenched centuries ago. This is the afterlife of slavery."

6. This is not to imply that homosexuality was, in some sense, apolitical prior to the 2000s. I use the term "politicization" to denote the process through which homosexuality has become a site of increasing social anxiety and alarm, a flashpoint or "symbolic target" (Weeks 2003:102) around which contestations over values, morality, sovereignty, and citizenship have converged.

7. According to Human Rights Watch (2021), the attendees were detained for twenty-two days, before being released on bail with charges of unlawful assembly. The case was subsequently dismissed due to lack of evidence.

8. Draft Promotion of Proper Human Sexual Rights and Ghanaian Family Values Bill 2021, Preamble.

9. Ashley Currier (2018:43) traces this shift in the Malawian context, noting that while homosexuality was politicized in countries such as Namibia, South Africa, Zambia, and Zimbabwe in the 1990s, this process occurred later in Malawi. This is also the case in Ghana.

10. Mark Gevisser (2020, 2021) dubs these emergent formations "the Pink Line," that is, "a geopolitical frontier in a new global culture war" (2021:7070).

11. The intersection of queer sexual orientation and vulnerability to HIV, alcohol and substance abuse, and poor health outcomes is also evident in South Africa, however, which has the most comprehensive set of legal rights and protections for LGBTI people on the continent.

12. I use the term "Afro-pessimism" here to refer to discourses that perpetuate the idea that "something is wrong with Africa," the genealogy of which dates back to the early colonial era (Louw and de B'béri 2011:337; see also Mudimbe 1988). While Afro-pessimist ways of talking and knowing about Africa are manifold and evolving, they are, according to Louw and de B'béri (2011:337), underpinned by the notion that "Africans are failing to live up to a set of criteria generated by Westerners."

13. Surya Munro et al. (2020:171) ascribe the heterogeneity of African gender and sexual norms to a number of factors, including "post-colonial and neo-colonial relations, local subjectivities, traditionalist patriarchies, and nationalist homophobias intertwining with human rights frameworks and activist interventions."

14. I am informed by Paul Farmer's definition of structural violence as essentially political economic in character, that is, as "social arrangements that put individuals and populations in harm's way. . . . The arrangements are structural because they are embedded in the political and economic organization of our social world; they are violent because they cause injury to people" (Farmer et al. 2006:1686). Political economic structures and conditions not only shape the uneven social and geographic distribution of extreme suffering, as is Farmer's primary concern, but also people's experiences of embodiment more generally, including forms of bodily pleasure (Altman 2001:2).

15. This introductory overview of the literature is intended to be illustrative rather than exhaustive and there are, of course, exceptions to these trends: see, for example, Peterson (2005) on the difference between "empirical" and "analytical" gender. I examine the diverse feminist political economy literature in more detail in chapters 1 and 3.

16. For scholarship that brings together Marxist political economy and queer approaches, see also Hennessy 2000; Floyd 2009; Liu 2015; Drucker 2015; Lewis 2016; Chitty 2020.

17. Methodologically the book is inspired by the rich ethnographic accounts of queer sexualities in West Africa produced by Dankwa (2021), in her work on erotic relationships between women in Ghana, and Rudi Gaudio (2009), in his monograph on "sexual outlaws" in the Hausa-speaking region of northern Nigeria. See also the doctoral theses of Matebeni (2012) and Thomann (2014) for ethnographic work on queer lives in South Africa and Côte d'Ivoire respectively.

18. As noted earlier, I am using "first wave" here to differentiate between the activists and organizations I studied in 2013–2015, who were operating at the nexus of HIV prevention and sexual rights advocacy in development, and the small but significant number of activist groups that have emerged since 2018, who are more explicitly focused on

LGBT+ rights. These newer groups include LGBT+ Rights Ghana, who were involved in setting up the LGBTQ+ community center in Accra that was shut down by the Ghanaian government in 2021.

19. The Akan, the largest ethnic group in Ghana, are estimated to represent 47.5 percent of the total population. After the Akan, the other largest ethnic groups are the Mole Dagbani (16.6 percent), the Ewe (13.9 percent), and the Ga-Adangbe (7.4 percent) (Ghana Statistical Service 2014:5).

20. In total, it is estimated that over eighty languages are spoken in Ghana, all belonging to branches of the Niger-Congo family (Guerini 2009:3; Kropp Dakubu 1997:6).

21. The presence of queer networks in and around Jamestown and central Accra, however, is well documented (see, for example, O'Mara 2007; Otu 2022).

22. An "outdooring" is a ceremonial event customary among the Ga, Akan, and Ewe ethnic groups in Ghana, in which a newborn child (usually on the eighth day after birth) is "introduced" to its family and the wider community (Adjah 2011:1).

23. I am conscious that this deployment of "Africa" may seem to imply a sense of homogeneity, or, more worryingly, to evoke colonial ideas of a single, essentialized "Africa." As Neville Hoad (2007:xv) points out, "Africa" is multivalent; its meanings are "contested and palimpsestic." In light of this, I follow Sylvia Tamale (2011) in employing Africa as a specific framing to highlight some of the similarities (and differences) in historical conditions across West, Central, East and southern Africa and to explore their relationship with formations of sexuality. These formations are, as Tamale puts it, deeply inscribed by "forces of colonialism, imperialism, globalization, capitalism, and fundamentalism" (2011:1).

24. The title of Matebeni's paper is a reference to Binyavanga Wainaina's influential parody essay, 'How to Write about Africa', first published in 2005. Wainaina (2019 [2005]) writes, "Always end your book with Nelson Mandela saying something about rainbows or renaissances. Because you care."

25. I discuss the historical, material, and cultural origins of "homosexuality" as a category of sexual difference in detail in Chapter 2.

26. David Halperin (1995:56), for example, describes "the ability of 'queer' to define (homo)sexual identity oppositionally and relationally but not necessarily substantively, not as a positivity but as a positionality, not as a thing, but as a resistance to the norm."

27. Roderick Ferguson's (2004) "queer of colour critique" similarly corrects the underdevelopment of race—and processes of racialization—as a key axis within formations of hetero- and homonormativity. Ferguson (2004) refers to this concept specifically as "racialized heteronormativity."

28. This scholarship has also documented how the politicization of homosexuality has reshaped indigenous language and naming practices in Ghana. According to Dankwa (2009), for example, the indigenous idiom *supi*, widely used to refer to erotic practices and relations between women, has become politically charged in the contemporary juncture, notably through its discursive association with Western constructs of lesbianism (thus sometimes becoming "*sup-supi* lesbianism"). A number of my research participants

highlighted a similar shift in popular understandings of the term *kwadwo basia*, which originates from the Akan name *Kwadwo*, meaning "Monday born," and *basia*, meaning feminine or ladylike. *Kwadwo basia* is a multivalent term that can be tied to gender, sexuality, identity, and humor and, according to William Banks (2013), has historically been used to refer to a feminine-presenting man or a man who dresses in women's clothing. However, the politicization of homosexuality since the 2000s has similarly worked to politicize *Kwadwo basia*, with the meaning of the term shifting from notions of gender expression to connote sexual orientation. As a result, it has been used in an increasingly derogative and stigmatizing way toward feminine-presenting (queer) men.

29. The value of defining queer as "anti-normative" and linking queerness to normativity in oppositional terms has been debated elsewhere by queer scholars (Wiegman and Wilson 2015; Hendriks 2021). Drawing on ethnographic research with self-identified "effeminate" men in the Democratic Republic of Congo, for example, Hendriks (2021) shows how his interlocuters "played into" rather than opposed dominant sexual and gender norms, notably as a means of seduction. In light of this, he argues that queerness is a "potential of normativity, rather than an opposition to it" (Hendriks 2021:399).

CHAPTER 1

1. Conversely, state laws may also provide certain rights and protections to queer populations, for example, through the passage of equal marriage laws for gay and lesbian couples or through the provision of protections from discrimination on the grounds of sexual orientation and gender identity.

2. I am using Onur Ulas Ince's conceptualization of "colonial capitalism" here as a means to highlight the central role of the (British) colonial empire in the emergence of capitalism. According to Ince (2018:4), colonial capitalism grasps "capitalist relations as having developed in and through colonial networks of commodities, peoples, ideas, and practices, which formed a planetary web of value chains connecting multiple and heterogeneous sites of production across oceanic distances." See also Ossome 2021 and Tamale 2020 for deployments of this concept within African political economy.

3. Importantly, however, formations of heteronormativity are also shifting and contingent, with dominant family-forms and models of intimacy and kinship transforming over time, in relation to broader processes of political economic change (Hennessy 2000; Duggan 2002; Eng 2010; Drucker 2015). This means that shifts in the social relations of production and reproduction essentially shape and reshape the limits and (im)possibilities of sexual freedom and repression (Sears 2017; Valocchi 2017).

4. Scholars have also drawn attention to the emergence of "homonormativity" in the neoliberal era, in which certain queer subjects—married, procreative, monogamous—have been assimilated into the nation-state, especially in Europe and North America (Duggan 2002). While I explore how homonormativity operates through structures of global governance and development processes, at the state level, I focus primarily on heteronormativity since that is the most salient to the domestic Ghanaian context.

5. Faced with both an economic crisis and a "crisis of hegemony" in the 1970s, Hall (1978) argues, the British state turned toward law and order as a key means of "policing the crisis." This shift was justified by racialized fears over rises in muggings and crime rates.

6. This speaks to the broader importance of connecting the cultural to the economic in understanding the materiality of sex and gender. As Rosemary Hennessy (2000:33) usefully puts it, this means attending to "the material relationship between the discourses by which we make the world intelligible and the structures of accumulation and labor on which capitalism irrevocably depends."

7. The Cameron controversy is not the only time that Western leaders have attempted to intervene in the governance of LGBTI rights in Ghana. In March 2023, US vice president Kamala Harris visited Ghana and, during a joint press conference with President Akufo-Addo, stated: "I feel very strongly about the importance of supporting the freedom and supporting the fighting for equality among all people, and that all people be treated equally. . . . I will also say that this [LGBTI rights] is an issue that we consider and I consider to be a human rights issue, and that will not change." Harris's intervention was criticized by Speaker of parliament, Alban Bagbin, a supporter of the anti-LGBTQ+ bill, who stated: "These things should not be tolerated, that is undemocratic" (Sahara Reporters 2023).

8. Altman's (1997) landmark paper "Global Gaze / Global Gays" theorized the mobility of Western forms of sexual subjectivity in Southeast Asia in relation to shifting global patterns of affluence and the new opportunities this creates for queer consumption, sometimes referred to as the "pink economy" (see also Binnie 2004). In Ghana, the concept of a gay consumer culture is less salient than in countries like the Philippines or Indonesia, since there is no comparable middle-class gay commercial "scene," even in cities like Accra. As per Altman's argument, this can be explained by the relative climate of intolerance toward LGBTI politics and queer communities in Ghana, and, I would add, by the highly uneven patterns of development that characterize the contemporary Ghanaian state.

9. In terms of this book, much of the analysis draws on evidence from anglophone Africa, given the commonalities with Ghana in terms of colonial inheritance. Extending this type of political economy analysis into parts of francophone and lusophone Africa would therefore be a fruitful future direction of research.

10. Unlike other African penal codes inherited from the British, the Ghanaian code defines "unnatural carnal knowledge" as the lesser criminal offence of "misdemeanor." It is also differs from other British-imposed codes in that it is not directly derived from the Indian Penal Code, but is understood to have originated from a draft code intended for Jamaica, formulated by the British jurist R. S. Wright (Human Rights Watch 2008:6).

11. As this suggests, the Constitution of Ghana does not provide any protections on the basis of sexual orientation or gender identity. It does, however, enshrine protection from discrimination on the grounds of "gender, race, colour, ethnic origin, religion, creed or social or economic status" (Article 17, Constitution of Ghana 1992).

12. One example of this from Ghana is "friendship marriage" among the Nzema of southern Ghana, which troubles the idea that precolonial Ghana was "heterosexual" (Dankwa 2021; Otu 2022).

13. See also Stoler 2002 and Epprecht 2005 on the impact of Christian missionary propaganda concerning sexual deviancy and propriety on understandings of queer sexualities in a number of African countries.

14. African Pentecostalism (also referred to here as Pentecostal-Charismatic Christianity) comprises a diverse group of churches and denominations that are pneumatic in orientation, i.e., that attribute a central role to the "pneuma" or Holy Spirit (Wariboko 2017:1). It is typically understood to comprise three primary types of movement: African-initiated/independent churches; churches that were set up in Africa by Western Pentecostal denominations; and neo-Pentecostal or charismatic churches.

15. David Paternotte (2020) argues that scholars should abandon the concept of "backlash" when it comes to analysing contemporary anti-LGBTI and anti-gender mobilizations, since it focuses attention primarily on the immediate objects under attack, rather than on how such attacks constitute "a wider project, which strives to establish a new political—less liberal and less democratic—order". I agree with Paternotte's overarching point, though I have, at times, chosen to use the term backlash to capture dynamics within the Ghanaian context, notably where the activities of queer and/or HIV activists (or purported activities of activists) have elicited strong "counter-offensives" from the state, religious institutions, or the media (as was the case with the "homoconference" controversy of 2006, for example).

16. President Mills's successor, John Dramani Mahama, initially stayed quiet on the issue of homosexuality during his presidency, which began in 2012. On a visit to the United States in 2013, for example, Mahama avoided answering any questions regarding his position on LGBTI rights (Ehrman-Dupre 2013). He also remained taciturn in the face of criticism over his appointment of Nana Oye Lithur—a well-known human rights lawyer and outspoken defender of LGBTI people in Ghana—to serve as a government minister. As dissent within his own party grew, however, the president clarified his position on homosexuality, stating that "the laws of Ghana are very clear on, appall, and criminalise homosexuality" (GhanaWeb 2013).

17. To date, the president has not publicly confirmed what he would do if the bill were passed by parliament, only calling for the debate to be held in a "civil" manner (Reuters 2021). While the lead sponsor of the bill, Sam George MP, and the majority of other sponsors are from the National Democratic Congress, it enjoys considerable cross-party support. In this sense, its significance includes and extends beyond party politics.

18. This is a rise from 28.3 percent of the population in 2010. Islam is the second largest affiliation, at 19.7 percent, followed by Protestant (17.4 percent) and Catholic (10 percent). Only 1.1 percent of the population said they had no religious affiliation (GSS 2022). This breakdown should be interpreted in the context of a broader "charismatization" of mainline Christianity in Ghana and West Africa, whereby mainline churches

have increasingly adopted the ethos, spiritual discourses, and style of Pentecostal-Christianity, in response to its surging popularity (Adogame 2013).

19. The regional conference was co-organized by Family Renaissance International (Ghana), CitizenGo (Kenya), and Family Watch International (United States), and lists attendees that include government officials, the media, academia, religious and traditional bodies, civil societies, NGOs, and interest groups (Catholic Secretariat of Nigeria 2019). A report by the European Parliamentary Forum for Sexual and Reproductive Rights (Datta 2021) identifies CitizenGo, Family Watch International, and the WCF among fifty-four key "anti-gender" funders and organizations operating globally since 2009.

CHAPTER 2

1. This HIV-driven trajectory is understood to characterize much of the African continent, with the exception of southern African countries such as South Africa and Zimbabwe, where activists began setting out strident calls for gay and lesbian rights in the 1980s (Gevisser and Cameron 1995; Epprecht 2011; see also Edwards and Epprecht 2020 on the history of working-class sexualities in South Africa).

2. Key populations are groups of people who are at higher risk of contracting HIV and who frequently lack access to services (UNAIDS 2015). The population groups are not always defined consistently but in Ghana are understood to include MSM, sex workers, people who inject drugs, and on remand prisoners (Ghana AIDS Commission 2017a).

3. This refers to a move from a "general population paradigm" in Ghana (that assumes a low-level generalized heterosexual epidemic) to a "key populations paradigm" (that recognizes the existence of a concentrated epidemic among certain sociodemographic groups, namely female sex workers and MSM) (Gyamerah 2021).

4. I am using "sexual minority rights" here as opposed to LGBTI rights, since this reflects the preferred terminology within international policy and legal spheres. See the introduction for a critique of this minoritarian framing of rights.

5. In a 2014 review of the policies and practices on LGBTI rights/SOGI among the twelve largest development agencies and Development Assistance Committee members, six agencies had incorporated LGBTI rights or SOGI into their strategic policy and/or had a specific policy about LGBTI rights and development, and ten agencies had leaders who had made public statements about LGBTI rights or SOGI (Bergenfield and Miller 2014).

6. See USAID 2014, "LGBTI Vision for Action."

7. DFID's 2014 Ghana Operational Plan, on the other hand, makes no reference to LGBTI rights.

8. HIV prevalence among the general population in Ghana was estimated at 1.7 per cent in 2018 (UNAIDS 2018). According to the most recently available statistics (from 2017), the prevalence among MSM in Ghana was estimated at 18.1 percent (Ghana AIDS Commission 2017b).

9. The Gay and Lesbian Association of Ghana, occasionally referenced in the academic literature on queer sexualities in Ghana (O'Mara 2007), operates more as a pseudonymized umbrella group when activists wish to speak out publicly. The queer women's group Sister to Sister, which was at one time connected to CEPEHRG, was no longer in operation at the time of my research.

10. This list is not meant to be exhaustive, rather to provide an overview of some of the key actors involved in what I term the first wave of queer activism in Ghana. There are also, for example, a number of other organizations involved exclusively in HIV prevention and sexual health service provision, including for MSM.

11. Unlike some other African countries where Pride events have emerged over the past five years, such as Malawi and Uganda, these events were not public protests/parades, but rather took place behind closed doors with a select group of invitees, for example, at the US and Dutch Embassies in Accra.

12. See Banks et al. 2015 for a discussion of these trends as characteristic of NGO-ization.

13. "We are not one" here means "We are not *sasso*/queer."

14. Godfried Asante (2022: 355) similarly observes how NGOs reinforce class hierarchies in his study of three LGBTI rights organizations in Ghana. He also notes that among some *sassoi*, "Classy" has become a type of identity performance, which is defined by the "co-constitution of the colonial Christian notion of masculinity, infused with western mediated forms of gay culture centred on fashion and style, enacted through a sexual politics based on invisibility". While I did not encounter this particular "glocalized" (Asante 2022) facet of queer sexual and class politics during my research, Asante's findings both resonate with and further illustrate the transformative impacts of NGO-ization on queer politics in this context. The complex and contradictory effects of HIV prevention and other sexual health rights initiatives on peer educators' subjective and embodied practices are explored in detail in Chapter 4.

15. Notions of "professionalization" and "capacity-building" also contain implicit assumptions about the (Western) location of knowledge and expertise, which are reproductive of neocolonial power relations.

16. Rodriguez (2019:108) refers to the latter practice as learning the "transnational language of human rights"; i.e., it is one of the practices through which queer African activists make themselves legible to pre-existing external structures, here in terms of development agendas and funding mechanisms.

17. CEPEHRG staff members also liaise with a small number of "friendly" government, donor, and civil society actors on HIV prevention efforts for KPs, for example, by attending working groups and by acting as a mouthpiece for and conduit of information to Accra's MSM networks.

18. Prince Macdonald is a pseudonym adopted by the activist for public campaigning and media appearances. For a detailed analyses of the "homoconference" panic see Dankwa 2021 and Essien and Aderinto 2006.

19. The Ugandan government's notorious "Anti-Homosexuality Bill," first intro-

duced in 2009, sought to outlaw gay marriage and "homosexual propaganda," and impose the death penalty for "aggravated homosexuality" (Nyanzi and Karamagi 2015). The bill was widely condemned by activists, civil society groups, and development organizations (Ssebaggala 2011). In 2013, a newer version of the bill was passed by the Ugandan parliament that reduced the penalty to life imprisonment, as part of the Anti-Homosexuality Act 2014. Even closer to home for Ghanaian activists, Nigeria has also moved to strengthen its anti-homosexuality legislation, through the Same-Sex Marriage Prohibition Act 2014. This law includes a raft of repressive measures targeted at queer individuals, including the prohibition of, and a prison sentence for participation in, "gay clubs, societies and organizations" (Carroll and Itaborahy 2015:61).

20. According to Martínez et al. (2021:94), this shift in rhetoric has a legitimating purpose, in that it allows groups like the NCPHSRFV "to speak a secular language that complements their religious narrative and positions their anti-LGBT rhetoric in a positive light."

CHAPTER 3

1. *Chalewɔte*, also referred to as "slippers," are the equivalent of flip-flops in UK English. The term comes from *chale* (or *chalé*), a colloquial word meaning "friend," and the Ga phrase *wɔte* ("Let's go"). Anecdotally, I was told that they were given the name *chalewɔte* because they are the footwear you put on when someone asks you to leave the house in a hurry.

2. Approximate to "They threw me out" in UK English.

3. See Biruk and Trapence 2017 for an important exception that looks at some of the risks faced by peer educators working for an LGBTI organization in Malawi.

4. Beyond peer education, many research participants were engaged in "feminized" jobs within the informal sector, such as hairdressing, food preparation, makeup artistry, and event planning. This reflected the difficulty they encountered in securing jobs in more formal and/or masculinized sectors of the Ghanaian economy, which acted as a serious constraint on their ability to generate income. Indeed, despite the widely noted inadequacy of the monthly stipend, it was clear that for a number of peer educators this was a crucial and—at times solitary—source of income, as Kofi explained: "The money is too small. But sometimes it is all you have."

5. One important exception to this trend is Shana Ye's (2021) study of queer men's intimate labor in the HIV/AIDS industry in China. Ye (2021:1788) links this economy to transnational labor regimes that (re)produce workers' precarity, which she argues are structurally sexualized in character. This chapter shares Ye's concern for the microlevel impacts of HIV interventions and their social reproductive dynamics, but explores this using an alternative approach, namely by examining MSM peer education in relation to development discourse on "empowerment," forms of gendered and racialized labor, and the crisis of social reproduction.

6. For a discussion of PRSPs in Ghana, see Crawford and Abdulai 2009.

7. In terms of healthcare in Ghana, the state has sought, for example, to extend the

coverage of national services through the introduction of the National Health Insurance Scheme in 2003, which, although still essentially privatized, replaced up-front payment with a nationalized scheme of health insurance (Abukari et al. 2015).

8. Some peer educators also reported being verbally abused by their peers, for example, in instances where the peer educator had encouraged an individual to get tested and he received a positive diagnosis for HIV.

CHAPTER 4

1. See Banks 2011 for an account of the idiomatic meanings of "sweetness" in relation to *sasso* sexual initiation practices—or *ntetee*—in Ghana.

2. This is not to imply that these were the only issues identified by activists as important. Other issues such as housing and freedom of assembly, association, and expression were also frequently mentioned by community and NGO-based activists. In identifying these four key issues, I have taken into account the most common ways in which activists expressed, conceptualized, and emphasized their political priorities, alongside their existing political practices, discussed in the second part of this chapter.

3. "Skirmish" is used in a similar way to "sashay," i.e., to walk/behave in an feminine manner, for example, through exaggerated movements of the hips.

4. When I first began my research in the early 2010s, I was surprised by the scale and visibility of some of the queer events and parties I was invited to attend in Accra. According to activists, however, these events had been toned down since the Jamestown incident, and were increasingly organized with a much stronger concern for security and privacy.

5. A study in Kenya and South Africa found, for example, higher levels of depression, anxiety, suicidality, and substance use among LGBTI individuals than among the general population (Müeller and Daskilewicz 2018).

6. These Pride events were not marches, but rather took place behind closed doors at the US Embassy in Accra. Due to fears over security, HRAC compiled an invite-only guest list of predominantly men working in or for LGBTI/HIV organizations.

7. Tamale is a large city in the northern region of Ghana.

8. Although Atu does not elaborate on the exact character of these arrangements, this type of transactional relationship can have significant implications for queer men's safety and well-being, particularly in terms of associated economic-, age-, and other power-related disparities and increased risk of HIV infection (Masvawure et al. 2015).

9. In light of this, Edward wanted to see Ghana's formal LGBTI/MSM organizations at least address the issue of decriminalization. He noted: "The unnatural knowledge law, that law, if it could be removed it would really help, because people are committing abuses, discriminating against us, violating our rights, assaulting us. The police in particular are using that to violate our rights."

10. "This community" refers to Jamestown.

11. The principles express rights in relation to the protected characteristics of sexual orientation and gender identity: for example, Principle 12, the right to work, stipulates

that "everyone has the right to decent and productive work, to just and favourable conditions of work and to protection against unemployment, without discrimination on the basis of sexual orientation or gender identity" (Yogyakarta Principles 2019).

CONCLUSION

1. These are detailed in Articles 162 and 165 of the Kenyan penal code respectively.

2. *Amicus curiae* refers to someone who is not a party to the case but assists the court by offering information, expertise or insight that may be relevant.

3. The Kenyan ruling in particular was seen as a setback since it followed a number of more positive outcomes for activists in the country, including a successful legal challenge to a government-imposed ban that prohibited the group, Transgender Education and Advocacy, from registering as a NGO in 2014, and a High Court ruling that allowed the trans activist, Audrey Mbugua, to officially change the name on her high school certificate, also in 2014 (BBC 2014).

4. Blantari's candor may seem surprising, given the key role of the Ghana Police Service in upholding and perpetrating politicized homophobia. While he is no doubt professionally isolated in his views, his comments and positioning also reflect the fundamentally contested character of queer sexual politics in the contemporary Ghanaian context and how this plays out in dynamic relation to the activities of NGOs and the HIV epidemic.

5. For the full statement see Appendix B.

6. Feminist scholars have long called for studies of global capitalism to centralize body politics (e.g., Youngs 2000; Federici 2004; Rioux 2015; Smith 2012, 2018; Hozić 2021). "Follow the bodies", Aida Hozić (2021:194) writes powerfully, "not just the money or the states and the deadly liberal silences over torture, genocides and wars would quickly turn into loud screams."

7. Given the problems associated with vertically structured, professionalized LGBTI/HIV NGOs in Ghana (as set out in Chapter 3), I would subscribe to an alternative, horizontal understanding of solidarity, premised on "mutuality, accountability, and the recognition of common interests as the basis for relationships among diverse communities" (Mohanty 2003:7).

8. Natalie Oswin (2007), for example, uses the Fraser-Butler debate to frame a historical analysis of the shifting politics of the South African organization, the National Coalition for Gay and Lesbian Equality.

9. See Appendix C for full statement.

BIBLIOGRAPHY

Abara, W. E., and Garba, I. (2017). HIV epidemic and human rights among men who have sex with men in sub-Saharan Africa: Implications for HIV prevention, care, and surveillance. *Global Public Health* 12 (4), 469–82. https://doi.org/10.1080/1744 1692.2015.1094107

Abukari, Z., Kuyini, A. B., and Mohammed, A. K. (2015). Education and health care policies in Ghana: Examining the prospects and challenges of recent provisions. *Sage Open* 5 (4), 1–11.

Adebanjo, A. T. (2015). Culture, morality and the law: Nigeria's anti-gay law in perspective. *International Journal of Discrimination and the Law* 15 (4), 256–70.

Adebajo, S. B., Eluwa, G. I., Allman, D., Myers, T., and Ahonsi, B. A. (2012). Prevalence of internalized homophobia and HIV associated risks among men who have sex with men in Nigeria. *African Journal of Reproductive Health* 16 (4), 21–28.

Adjah, O. (2011). What is in a name? Ghanaian personal names as information sources. *Journal of the African Studies Association of the UK* 117, 3–17.

Adjepong, A. (2021). *Afropolitan Projects: Redefining Blackness, Sexualities and Culture from Houston to Accra*. Chapel Hill: University of North Carolina Press.

Adogame, A. (2013). Reconfiguring the global religious economy: The role of African Pentecostalism. In D. Miller, K. Sargeant, and R. Flory (eds.), *Spirit and Power: The Growth and Global Impact of Pentecostalism*, 32–42. Oxford University Press.

Adomako Ampofo, A. (2001). "When men speak women listen": Gender socialisation and young adolescents' attitudes to sexual and reproductive issues. *African Journal of Reproductive Health* 5 (3), 196–212.

Adomako Ampofo, A., and Boateng, J. (2011). Multiple meanings of manhood in Ghana. In S. Tamale (ed.), *African Sexualities: A Reader*, 420–36. Oxford: Pambazuka Press.

Adomako Ampofo, A., Okyerefo, M., and Pervarah, M. (2009). Phallic competence: Fatherhood and the making of men in Ghana. *Culture, Society and Masculinity* 1 (1), 59–78.

African Lesbian, Gay, Bisexual, Transgender and Intersex (LGBTI) Manifesto/Declaration. (2010). Nairobi. https://blacklooks.org/2011/05/african-lgbti-manifestodeclaration/ (accessed January 31, 2020).

Agathangelou, A. (2006). *The Global Political Economy of Sex: Desire, Violence, and Insecurity in Mediterranean Nation States*. Basingstoke: Palgrave Macmillan.

Agyemang, F. O., Asamoah, P. K. B., and Obodai, J. (2018). Changing family systems in Ghana and its effects on access to urban rental housing: A study of the Offinso Municipality. *Journal of Housing and the Built Environment* 33, 893–916.

Akanji, O., and Epprecht, M. (2013). Human rights challenge in Africa: Sexual minority rights and the African Charter on Human and Peoples' Rights. In S. N. Nyeck and M. Epprecht (eds.), *Sexual Diversity in Africa: Politics, Theory, and Citizenship*, 19–36. Montreal: McGill-Queen's University Press.

Akinwotu, A. (2021). Ghanaian LGBTQ+ centre closes after threats and abuse. *The Guardian*, 25 February. https://www.theguardian.com/global-development/2021/feb/25/lgbtq-ghanaians-under-threatafter-backlash-against-new-support-centre

Alexander, M. J. (1994). Not just (any) body can be a citizen: The politics of law, sexuality and postcoloniality in Trinidad and Tobago and the Bahamas. *Feminist Review* 48 (1), 5–23. https://doi.org/10.1057/fr.1994.39

Alexander, M. J. (2005). *Pedagogies of Crossing: Meditations on Feminism, Sexual Politics, Memory and the Sacred*. Durham, NC: Duke University Press.

Ali, H., Amoyaw, F., Baden, D., Durand, L., Bronson, M., Kim, A., Grant-Greene, Y., Imtiaz, R., and Swaminathan, M. (2019). Ghana's HIV epidemic and PEPFAR's contribution towards epidemic control. *Ghana Medical Journal* 53 (1), 59–62.

Altman, D. (1996). Rupture or continuity? The internationalization of gay identities. *Social Text*, no. 48, 77–94.

Altman, D. (1997). Global gaze / global gays. *GLQ: A Journal of Lesbian and Gay Studies* 3 (4), 417–36.

Altman, D. (2001). *Global Sex*. Chicago: University of Chicago Press.

Amadiume, I. (1987). *Male Daughters, Female Husbands: Gender and Sex in an African Society*. London: Zed Books.

Amin, S. (1972). Underdevelopment and dependence in Black Africa: Origins and Contemporary forms. *Journal of Modern African Studies* 10 (4), 503–24. http://www.jstor.org/stable/160011

Andrucki, M. (2017). Queering social reproduction, or, How queers save the city. *Society + Space*, October 31. https://www.societyandspace.org/articles/queering-social-reproduction-or-how-queers-save-the-city

Arat-Koc, S. (2006). Whose social reproduction? Transnational motherhood and challenges to feminist political economy. In K. Bezanson and M. Luxton (eds.), *Social Reproduction: Feminist Political Economy Challenges Neoliberalism*, 75–92. Montreal: McGill-Queen's University Press.

Armisen, M. (2016). We exist: Mapping LGBTQ organizing in West Africa. Ouagadougou: Queer African Youth Network.

Arnfred, S. (2004). "African sexuality" / sexuality in Africa: Tales and silences. In S. Arnfred (ed.), *Re-thinking Sexualities in Africa*, 59–78. Uppsala: Nordic Africa Institute.

Arruzza, C., Bhattacharya, T., and Fraser, N. (2019). *Feminism for the 99%: A Manifesto*. London: Verso Books.

Aryeetey, E. and Fenny, A. (2017). Economic growth in Ghana: Trends and structure, 1960–2014. In E. Aryeetey and R. Kanbur (eds.), *The Economy of Ghana Sixty Years after Independence*, 45–65. Oxford University Press.

Asante, G. (2020). Anti-LGBT violence and the ambivalent (colonial) discourses of Ghanaian Pentecostalist-Charismatic church leaders. *Howard Journal of Communications* 31 (1), 20–34. https://doi.org/10.1080/10646175.2019.1590255

Asante, G. (2022). "They just need to empower themselves:" reproducing queer (neo) *liberalism* in LGBTS empowerment discourses of representatives of LGBTS Human Rights NGOs in Ghana, *Communication and Critical/Cultural Studies*, 19 (4), 344–62, https://doi.org/10.1080/14791420.2022.2113109

Attipoe, D. (2004). Revealing the Pandora Box or playing the ostrich? A situational appraisal of men having sex with men in the Accra metropolitan area and its environs—Ghana. Unpublished. Accra: West Africa Project to Combat HIV/AIDS and STIs.

Awondo, P. (2010). The politicisation of sexuality and rise of homosexual movements in post-colonial Cameroon. *Review of African Political Economy* 37 (125), 315–28.

Awondo, P., Geschiere, P., and Reid, G. (2012). Homophobic Africa? Toward a more nuanced view. *African Studies Review* 55 (3), 145–68.

Ayen, N. (1998). West African homoeroticism: West African men who have sex with men. In S. Murray and W. Roscoe (eds.), *Boy-Wives and Female Husbands: Studies in African Homosexualities*, 129–41. New York: Palgrave Macmillan.

Bair, J. (2010). On Difference and Capital: Gender and the Globalization of Production. *Signs* 36 (1), 203–26. https://doi.org/10.1086/652912

Bakker, I. (2007). Social reproduction and the constitution of a gendered political economy. *New Political Economy* 12 (4), 541–56. https://doi.org/10.1080/13563460701661561

Bakker, I., and Gill, S. (eds.). (2003). *Power, Production and Social Reproduction: Human In/security in the Global Political Economy*. Basingstoke: Palgrave Macmillan.

Banks, N., Hulme, D., and Edwards, M. (2015). NGOs, states, and donors revisited: Still too close for comfort? *World Development* 66, 707–18.

Banks, W. (2011). "This thing is sweet": Nteteε and the reconfiguration of sexual subjectivity in post-colonial Ghana. *Ghana Studies*, 14, 265–69.

Banks, W. (2013). Queering Ghana: sexuality, community, and the struggle for cultural belonging in an African nation. PhD diss., Wayne State University.

Baral, S., Trapence, G., Motimedi, F., Umar, E., Iipinge, S., Dausadb, F., and Beyrer, C. (2009). HIV prevalence, risks for HIV infection, and human rights among men who have sex with men (MSM) in Malawi, Namibia, and Botswana. *PLoS ONE* 4 (3), e4997.

Batliwala, S. (2007). Taking the power out of empowerment—an experiential account. *Development in Practice* 17 (4–5), 557–65. https://doi.org/10.1080/09614520701469559

Bawa, S. (2019). Christianity, tradition, and gender inequality in postcolonial Ghana.

African Geographical Review 38 (1), 54–66. https://doi.org/10.1080/19376812.2017 .1286245

BBC. (2006). Ghanaian gay conference banned. BBC, September 1. http://news.bbc.co .uk/1/hi/world/africa/5305658.stm

BBC. (2011). Cameron threat to dock some UK aid to anti-gay nations. BBC, October 30. http://www.bbc.co.uk/news/uk-15511081

BBC. (2014). Kenya court victory for transgender activist Audrey Mbugua. BBC, October 7. https://www.bbc.co.uk/news/world-africa-29519881

Bedford, K. (2005). Loving to straighten out development: Sexuality and "ethnodevelopment" in the World Bank's Ecuadorian lending. *Feminist Legal Studies* 13 (3), 295–322.

Bedford, K. (2009). *Developing Partnerships: Gender, Sexuality, and the Reformed World Bank*. Minneapolis: University of Minnesota Press.

Bedford, K. (2016). Bingo regulation and the feminist political economy of everyday gambling: In search of the anti-heroic. *Globalizations* 13 (6), 801–14. https://doi.org /10.1080/14747731.2016.1164981

Behar, R. (1996). *The Vulnerable Observer: Anthropology That Breaks Your Heart*. Boston: Beacon Press.

Benería, L. (2003). *Gender, Development, and Globalization*. New York: Routledge.

Berg, H. (2021). *Porn Work: Sex, Labor, and Late Capitalism*. Chapel Hill: University of North
Carolina Press.

Bergenfield, R., and Miller, A. M. (2014). Queering international development? An examination of new "LGBT rights" rhetoric, policy, and programming among international development agencies. *SSRN Electronic Journal*, October, 1–18. https://doi .org/10.2139/ssrn.2507515

Bergeron, S. (2010). Querying economics' straight path to development: Household models reconsidered. In A. Lind (ed.), *Development, Sexual Rights and Global Governance*, 54–64. Abingdon: Routledge.

Bergeron, S. (2011). Economics, performativity, and social reproduction in global development. *Globalizations* 8 (2), 151–61. https://doi.org/10.1080/14747731.2010.493014

Bergeron, S., and Puri, J. (2012). Sexuality between state and class: An introduction. *Rethinking Marxism* 24 (4), 491–98. https://doi.org/10.1080/08935696.2012.711047

Berlant, L., and Warner, M. (1998). Sex in public. *Critical Inquiry* 24 (2), 547–66.

Beyrer, C. (2010). Global prevention of HIV infection for neglected populations: Men who have sex with men. *Clinical Infectious Diseases* 50(s3), S108–S113. https://doi.org /10.1086/651481

Beyrer, C. (2012). LGBTI Africa: A social justice movement emerges in the era of HIV. *Sahara Journal* 9 (3), 177–79. https://doi.org/10.1080/17290376.2012.743813

Beyrer, C., Baral, S. D., Van Griensven, F., Goodreau, S. M., Chariyalertsak, S., Wirtz, A. L., and Brookmeyer, R. (2012). Global epidemiology of HIV infection in men who have sex with men. *The Lancet* 380 (9839), 367–77. https://doi.org/10.1016/S0140-67 36(12)60821-6

Beyrer, C., Sullivan, P. S., Sanchez, J., Dowdy, D., Altman, D., Trapence, G., and Mayer, K. H. (2012). A call to action for comprehensive HIV services for men who have sex with men. *The Lancet* 380 (9839), 424–38. https://doi.org/10.1016/S0140-6736 (12)61022-8

Bezanson, K. and Luxton, M. (eds.) (2006) *Social Reproduction: Feminist Political Economy Challenges Neo-liberalism*. Montreal: McGill-Queen's University Press

Bhattacharyya, G. (2018). *Rethinking Racial Capitalism: Questions of Reproduction and Survival*. London: Rowman and Littlefield.

Bhattacharya, T. (2017). Introduction: Mapping social reproduction theory. In T. Bhattacharya (ed.), *Social Reproduction Theory: Remapping Class, Recentering Oppression*, 1–20. London: Pluto Press.

Binnie, J. (2004). *The Globalization of Sexuality*. London: Sage Publications.

Binnie, J. (2014). Neoliberalism, Class, Gender and Lesbian, Gay, Bisexual, Transgender and Queer Politics in Poland. *International Journal of Politics, Culture, and Society* 27 (2), 241–57. http://www.jstor.org/stable/24713315

Biruk, C. (2020). "Fake gays" in queer Africa: NGOs, metrics, and modes of (queer) theory. *GLQ: A Journal of Lesbian and Gay Studies* 26 (3), 477–502.

Biruk, C., and Trapence, G. (2018). Community engagement in an economy of harms: Reflections from an LGBTI-rights NGO in Malawi. *Critical Public Health* 28 (3), 340–51.

Bochow, A. (2008). Valentine's Day in Ghana: Youth, sex and secrets. In E. Alber, S. van der Geest, and S. Whyte (eds.), *Generations in Africa: Connections and Conflicts*, 333–56. Berlin: LIT Verlag.

Boellstorff, T. (2005). *The Gay Archipelago: Sexuality and Nation in Indonesia*. Princeton, NJ: Princeton University Press.

Boellstorff, T. (2007). *A Coincidence of Desires: Anthropology, Queer Studies, Indonesia*. Durham, NC: Duke University Press.

Boellstorff, T. (2011). But do not identify as gay: A proleptic genealogy of the MSM category. *Cultural Anthropology* 26 (2), 287–312.

Boellstorff, T. (2012). The politics of similitude: Global sexuality activism, ethnography, and the Western subject. *Trans-Scripts* 2, 22–39.

Boyce, P. (2007). "Conceiving kothis": Men who have sex with men in India and the cultural subject of HIV prevention. *Medical Anthropology* 26 (2), 175–203.

Boyce, P. (2014). Desirable rights: Same-sex sexual transformations, global flows and boundaries—in India and beyond. *Culture, Health and Sexuality* 16, 1–15.

Broqua, C. (2013). Male homosexuality in Bamako: A cross-cultural and cross-historical comparative perspective. In S. N. Nyeck and M. Epprecht (eds.), *Sexual Diversity in Africa: Politics, Theory, and Citizenship*, 208–24. Montreal: McGill-Queen's University Press.

Broqua, C. (2015). AIDS activism from north to global. In D. Paternotte and M. Tremblay (eds.), *The Ashgate Research Companion to Lesbian and Gay Activism*, 153–66. London: Routledge.

Brown, R. (2019). In historic shift, Botswana declares homosexuality is not a crime.

Christian Science Monitor, June 11, 2019. https://www.csmonitor.com/World/Africa /2019/0611/In-historic-shift-Botswana-declares-homosexuality-is-not-a-crime

Brown, W. (2003). Neo-liberalism and the end of liberal democracy. *Theory and Event* 7 (1). https://doi.org/10.1353/tae.2003.0020

Budhiraja, S., Fried, S. T., and Teixeira, A. (2010). Spelling it out: From alphabet soup to sexual rights and gender justice. In A. Lind (ed.), *Development, Sexual Rights and Global Governance*, 131–44. London: Routledge.

Butler, J. (1998). Merely cultural. *New Left Review* 227, 33–43. https://doi.org/10.2307/46 6744

Butler, J. (2004). *Undoing Gender*. London: Routledge.

Butler, J. (2021). Why is the idea of "gender" provoking backlash the world over? *The Guardian*, October 23, 2021. https://www.theguardian.com/us-news/commentisfree /2021/oct/23/judith-butler-gender-ideology-backlash

Campbell, C. and Mzaidume, Z. (2001). Grassroots participation, peer education, and HIV prevention by sex workers in South Africa. *American Journal of Public Health* 91 (12), 1978–86.

Castro, M. G., and Hallewell, L. (2016). Engendering powers in neoliberal times in Latin America: Reflections from the left on feminisms and feminisms. *Latin American Perspectives* 28 (6), 17–37.

Catholic Secretariat of Nigeria. (2019). *Report: World Congress of Families Regional Conference, Accra, Ghana 2019*. Church and Society Department of the Catholic Secretariat of Nigeria. https://fhl.csn-churchandsociety.org/world-congress-of-families -regional-conference-accra-ghana-2019-report/ (accessed May 17, 2023).

Chan, J. (2015). *Politics in the Corridor of Dying: AIDS Activism and Global Health Governance*. Baltimore: Johns Hopkins University Press.

Chant, S. (2008). The "feminisation of poverty" and the "feminisation" of anti-poverty programs: Room for revision? *Journal of Development Studies* 44 (2), 165–97. https:// doi.org/10.1080/00220380701789810

Chitty, C. 2020. *Sexual Hegemony: Statecraft, Sodomy, and Capital in the Rise of the World System*. Durham, NC: Duke University Press.

Choudry, A., and Kapoor, D. (eds.). (2013). *NGOization: Complicity, Contradictions and Prospects*. London: Zed Books.

Clark, G. (1999). Mothering, work, and gender in urban Asante ideology and practice. *American Anthropologist* 101 (4), 717–29.

Clarke, D. (2013). Twice removed: African invisibility in Western queer theory. In S. Ekine and H. Abbas (eds.), *Queer African Reader*, 173–85. Oxford: Pambazuka Press.

Clifford, J., and Marcus, G. E. (1986). *Writing Culture: The Poetics and Politics of Ethnography*. Berkeley: University of California Press.

Coalition Against Homophobia in Ghana. (2011). Press release on the British prime minister's "Homosexuality Threat" to Ghana from the Coalition against Homophobia in Ghana (CAHG). http://africanactivistarchive.blogspot.com/2011/11/lgbti-ac tivists-say-no-to-uk-prime.html (accessed January 31, 2020).

Cohen, C. J. (2005). Punks, bulldaggers, and welfare queens: The radical potential of queer politics? In P. E. Johnson and M. G. Henderson (eds.), *Black Queer Studies: A Critical Anthology*, 21–51. Durham, NC: Duke University Press.

Cook, M. (2014). *Queer Domesticities: Homosexuality and Home Life in Twentieth-Century London*. New York: Springer.

Cook, S., Sandfort, T., Nel, J., and Rich, E. (2013). Exploring the relationship between gender nonconformity and mental health among Black South African gay and bisexual men. *Archives of Sexual Behavior* 42 (3), 327–30. https://doi.org/10.1038/jid.2014.371

Cornwall, A. (2016). Women's empowerment: What works? *Journal of International Development* 28 (3), 342–59. https://doi.org/10.1002/jid.3210.

Cornwall, R. 1997. Queer Political Economy: The Social Articulation of Desire. In A. Gluckman and B. Reed (eds.), *Homo Economics: Capitalism, Community, and Lesbian and Gay Life*, 89–122. New York: Routledge.

Corrêa, S., Petchesky, R., and Parker, R. (2008). *Sexuality, Health and Human Rights*. London: Routledge.

Costa Santos, d. G., and Waites, M. (2019). Comparative colonialisms for queer analysis: Comparing British and Portuguese colonial legacies for same-sex sexualities and gender diversity in Africa—setting a transnational research agenda. *International Review of Sociology* 29 (2), 297–326. https://doi.org/10.1080/03906701.2019.1641277

Cotterill, J., and Pilling, D. (2019). Botswana court decriminalises homosexuality. *Financial Times*, June 11. https://www.ft.com/content/68a5d6ae-8c36-11e9-a1c1-51bf8f989972

Crawford, G., and Abdulai, A. G. (2009). The world bank and Ghana's poverty reduction strategies: Strengthening the state or consolidating neoliberalism? *Labor, Capital and Society* 42 (1–2), 82–115.

Crerar, P. (2018). Theresa May says she deeply regrets Britain's legacy of anti-gay laws. *Guardian Online*, April 17. https://www.theguardian.com/world/2018/apr/17/theresa-may-deeply-regrets-britain-legacy-anti-gay-laws-commonwealth-nations-urged-overhaul-legislation

Currier, A. (2010). The strategy of normalization in the South African LGBTI movement. *Mobilization* 15 (1), 45–62.

Currier, A. (2012). *Out in Africa: LGBTI Organizing in Namibia and South Africa*. Minneapolis: University of Minnesota Press.

Currier, A. (2015). Transgender invisibility in Namibian and South African LGBTI organizing. *Feminist Formations* 27 (1), 91–117.

Currier, A. (2016). Arrested solidarity: Obstacles to intermovement support for LGBTI rights in Malawi. *Women's Studies Quarterly* 42 (3), 146–63.

Currier, A. (2018). *Politicizing Sex in Contemporary Africa: Homophobia in Malawi*. Cambridge University Press.

Currier, A., and McKay, T. (2017). Pursuing social justice through public health: Gender and sexual diversity activism in Malawi. *Critical African Studies* 9 (1), 71–90.

Currier, A., and Migraine-George, T. (2016). Queer studies / African studies: An (im)possible transaction? *GLQ: A Journal of Lesbian and Gay Studies* 22 (2), 281–305.

Daily Graphic. (2011). 8,000 gays in 2 regions: Majority infected with HIV/AIDS. *Daily Graphic*, June 1. https://www.modernghana.com/news/331727/8000-homos-in-two-regions-majority-infected-with-hivaids.html

Daily Graphic. (2018). 3-day prayer crusade against same sex marriage scheduled for June 30. *Graphic Online*, June 6. https://www.graphic.com.gh/news/general-news/3-day-prayer-crusade-against-same-sex-marriage-scheduled-for-june-30.html

Daily Guide. (2013). Tamale residents chase gays. *Daily Guide*, August 24. http://www.ghanaweb.com/GhanaHomePage/NewsArchive/Tamale-residents-chase-gays-283508

Daily Guide. (2015a). Ghanaians must reject homosexuality—Rev. Dr. Nuakoh. *Daily Guide*, August 11. http://www.myjoyonline.com/news/2015/august-11th/ghanaians-must-reject-homosexuality-rev-dr-nuakoh.php

Daily Guide. (2015b). Owusu Bempah warns prez: "No gay marriage in Ghana." *Daily Guide*, July 9. http://www.ghanaweb.com/GhanaHomePage/NewsArchive/Owusu-Bempah-warns-Prez-No-Gay-marriage-in-Ghana-367462

Daily Guide. (2015c). Nima youth assault gay man. *Daily Guide*, August 17. http://www.ghanaweb.com/GhanaHomePage/crime/Nima-youth-assault-gay-man-375655

Dankwa, S. O. (2009). "It's a silent trade": Female same-sex intimacies in post-colonial Ghana. *Nordic Journal of Feminist and Gender Research* 17 (3), 192–205.

Dankwa, S. O. (2021). *Knowing Women: Same-Sex Intimacies, Gender, and Identity in Postcolonial Ghana*. Cambridge University Press.

Datta, N. (2021). *Tip of the Iceberg: Religious Extremist Funders against Human Rights for Sexuality and Reproductive Health in Europe 2009 – 2018*. Brussels: European Parliamentary Forum. https://www.epfweb.org/sites/default/files/2021-06/Tip%20of%20the%20Iceberg%20June%202021%20Final.pdf (accessed Jan 10, 2024).

Dave, S., Peter, T., Fogarty, C., Karatzas, N., Belinsky, N., and Pant Pai, N. (2019). Which community-based HIV initiatives are effective in achieving UNAIDS 90-90-90 targets? A systematic review and meta-analysis of evidence (2007–2018). *Plos One* 14 (7), e0219826.

Davis, A. (1981). *Women, Race and Class*. New York: Random House.

Davis, A. (2016). *Freedom Is a Constant Struggle: Ferguson, Palestine, and the Foundations of a Movement*. Chicago: Haymarket Press.

Deacon, G., and Lynch, G. (2013). Allowing Satan in? Moving toward a political economy of neo-Pentecostalism in Kenya. *Journal of Religion in Africa* 43, 108–30.

D'Emilio, J. (1993). Capitalism and gay identity. In H. Abelove, M. A. B. Barale, and D. Halperin (eds.), *The Lesbian and Gay Studies Reader*, 467–78. London: Routledge.

Department for International Development (DFID). (2014). Operational Plan 2011–2016 DFID Uganda. Department for International Development. https://assets.publishing.service.gov.uk/government/uploads/system/uploads/attachment_data/file/389293/Uganda.pdf (accessed May 17, 2023).

Dhawan, N., Engel, A., Govrin, J., Holzhey, C., and Woltersdorff, V. (eds.). (2015). *Global Justice and Desire: Queering Economy.* London: Routledge.

donortracker. (2023). Issue: Global health. https://donortracker.org/topics/globalhealth (accessed May 17, 2023).

Driskill, Q.-L. (2004). Stolen from our bodies: First Nations two-spirits / queers and the journey to a sovereign erotic. *Studies in American Indian Literatures* 16 (2), 50–64.

Drucker, P. (2009). Changing families and communities: An LGBT contribution to an alternative development path. *Development in Practice* 19 (7), 825–36. http://www.jstor.org/stable/27752137

Drucker, P. (2015). *Warped: Gay Normality and Queer Anti-capitalism.* Leiden: Brill.

Duggan, L. (2002). The new homonormativity: The sexual politics of neoliberalism. In R. Castronovo and D. D. Nelson (eds.), *Materializing Democracy: Toward a Revitalized Cultural Politics,* 175–94. Durham, NC: Duke University Press.

Duggan, L., and Kim, R. (2012). Preface: A new queer agenda. *SandF Online* 10 (1–2). http://sfonline.barnard.edu/a-new-queer-agenda/preface/

Dunne, P. (2012). LGBTI rights and the wrong way to give aid. *Harvard Kennedy School Review* 12, 66.

Edelman, L. (2004). *No Future: Queer Theory and the Death Drive.* Durham, NC: Duke University Press.

Edwards, I., and Epprecht, M. (2020). *Working Class Homosexuality in South African History: Voices from the Archive.* Cape Town: HSRC Press.

Ehrenreich B., Hochschild A. (2002). *Global Woman: Nannies, Maids, and Sex Workers in the New Economy.* New York: Henry Holt.

Ehrman-Dupre, J. (2013). Ghanaian president would rather not discuss gay marriage. *Towleroad,* October 4. http://www.towleroad.com/2013/10/ghanaian-president-visits-georgia-university-remains-silent-on-issue-of-gay-marriage/

Ekine, S., and Abbas, H. (eds.). (2013). *Queer African Reader.* Oxford: Pambazuka Press.

Elias, J., and Rai, S. (2019). Feminist everyday political economy: Space, time, and violence. *Review of International Studies* 45 (2), 201–20. https://doi.org/10.1017/S0260210518000323.

Elias, J., and Rethel, L. (2018). *The Everyday Political Economy of Southeast Asia.* Cambridge University Press.

Elias, J., and Roberts, A. (2016). Feminist global political economies of the everyday: From bananas to bingo. *Globalizations* 13 (6), 787–800. https://doi.org/10.1080/14747731.2016.1155797

Elias, J., and Roberts, A. (2018). *Handbook on the International Political Economy of Gender.* Cheltenham, UK: Edward Elgar.

Elson, D. (1992). From survival strategies to transformation strategies: Women's needs and structural adjustment. In L. Benería and S. Feldman (eds.), *Economic Crisis, Persistent Poverty and Women's Work,* 26–48. Boulder: Westview.

Elson, D. (1993). Gender-aware analysis and development economics. *Journal of International Development* 5, 237–47. https://doi.org/10.1002/jid.3380050214

Elson, D. (1999). Labor markets as gendered institutions: Equality, efficiency and empowerment issues. *World Development* 27 (3), 611–27. https://doi.org/10.1016/S0 305-750X(98)00147-8

Eng, D. (2010). *The Feeling of Kinship: Queer Liberalism and the Racialization of Intimacy*. Durham, NC: Duke University Press.

Eng, D., and Puar, J. (2020). Introduction: Left of queer. *Social Text* 2020 (4), 1–23.

Enloe, C. (2000). *Bananas, Beaches and Bases: Making Feminist Sense of International Politics*. Berkeley: University of California Press.

Epprecht, M. (2004). *Hungochani: The History of a Dissident Sexuality in Southern Africa*. Montreal: McGill-Queen's University Press.

Epprecht, M. (2005). Black skin, "cowboy" masculinity: A genealogy of homophobia in the African nationalist movement in Zimbabwe to 1983. *Culture, Health and Sexuality* 7 (3), 253–66. https://doi.org/10.1080/13691050410001730243

Epprecht, M. (2008). *Heterosexual Africa? The History of an Idea from the Age of Exploration to the Age of AIDS*. Athens: Ohio University Press; Scottsville: University of KwaZulu-Natal Press.

Epprecht, M. (2012). Sexual minorities, human rights and public health strategies in Africa. *African Affairs* 111 (March), 223–43. https://doi.org/10.1093/afraf/ads019

Epprecht, M. (2013). *Sexuality and Social Justice in Africa: Rethinking Homophobia and Forging Resistance*. London: Zed Books.

Essien, K., and Aderinto, S. (2009). "Cutting the head of the roaring monster": Homosexuality and repression in Africa. *African Study Monographs* 30 (3), 121–35.

Eveslage, B. (2015). Sexual health or rights? USAID-funded HIV/AIDS interventions for sexual minorities in Ghana. In J. Gideon and M. Liete (eds.), *Gender and Health Handbook*, 539–60. Cheltenham, UK: Edward Elgar.

Farmer, P. E, Nizeye, B., Stulac, S., and Keshavjee, S. (2006). Structural violence and clinical medicine. *PLoS Medicine* 3 (10), e449. https://doi.org/10.1371/journal.pmed.0030449

Faust, L., and Yaya, S. (2018). The effect of HIV educational interventions on HIV-related knowledge, condom use, and HIV incidence in sub-Saharan Africa: A systematic review and meta-analysis. *BMC Public Health* 18 (1), 1–14. https://doi.org/10.1186/s12889-018-6178-y

Fay, H., Baral, S. D., Trapence, G., et al. (2011). Stigma, health care access, and HIV knowledge among men who have sex with men in Malawi, Namibia, and Botswana. *AIDS and Behavior* 15 (2011), 1088–97. https://doi.org/10.1007/s10461-010-9861-2

Federici, S. (2004). *Caliban and the Witch: Women, the Body and Primitive Accumulation*. Brooklyn, NY: Autonomedia.

Feinberg, L. (1992). *Transgender Liberation: A Movement Whose Time Has Come*. New York: World View Forum Publishing.

Ferguson, R. A. (2004). *Aberrations in Black: Toward a Queer of Color Critique*. Minneapolis: University of Minnesota Press.

Ferguson, S. (2016). Intersectionality and social-reproduction feminisms: Toward an integrative ontology. *Historical Materialism* 24 (2), 38–60.

Ferguson, S. (2019). *Women and Work: Feminism, Labour, and Social Reproduction*. London: Pluto Press.

Fisher, J. (2015). "Does it work?"—work for whom? Britain and political conditionality since the Cold War. *World Development* 75, 13–25. https://doi.org/10.1016/j.worlddev.2014.12.005

Floyd, K. (2009). *The Reification of Desire: Toward a Queer Marxism*. Minneapolis: University of Minnesota Press.

Fortunati, L. (1995). *The arcane of reproduction: housework, prostitution, labor and capital*. Brooklyn, NY: Autonomedia.

Foucault, M. (1978). *History of Sexuality Volume I: The Will to Knowledge*. New York: Random House.

Fraser, N. (1997). *Justice Interruptus: Critical Reflections on the "Postsocialist" Condition*. New York: Routledge.

Fraser, N. (2016). Contradictions of capital and care. *New Left Review* 100, 99–117.

Fraser, N. (2022). *Cannibal Capitalism: How Our System Is Devouring Democracy, Care and the Planet—and What We Can Do about It*. London: Verso Books.

Frimpong, E. D. (2013). I will not promote homosexuality in Ghana—Nana Oye Lithur. *Graphic Online*, January 30. http://www.graphic.com.gh/news/general-news/i-will-not-promote-homosexuality-in-ghana-nana-oye-lithur.html

Gaudio, R. (2009). *Allah Made Us: Sexual Outlaws in an Islamic African City*. Malden, MA: Blackwell.

Gevisser, M. (2020). *The Pink Line: The World's Queer Frontiers*. London: Profile Books.

Gevisser, M. (2021). Response by the author. *Africa* 91 (4), 706–8. https://doi.org/10.1017/S0001972021000541

Gevisser, M., and Cameron, E. (2017). *Defiant Desire*. London: Routledge.

Ghana AIDS Commission. (2010). *National HIV and AIDS Strategic Plan: 2011–2015*. Accra: GAC.

Ghana AIDS Commission (2014). *Standard Operating Procedures for Implementing HIV Programs among Key Populations*. Accra: GAC.

Ghana AIDS Commission. (2016). *National HIV and AIDS Strategic Plan, 2016–2020*. Accra: GAC.

Ghana AIDS Commission. (2018). *Standard Operating Procedures for Implementing HIV Programs among Key Populations*. Accra: GAC.

Ghana AIDS Commission. (2017a). *Ghana AIDS Commission National and Sub-national HIV and AIDS Estimates and Projections 2017 Report*. Accra: GAC.

Ghana AIDS Commission. (2017b). *Ghana Men's Study II, 2017*. Accra: GAC.

Ghana Statistical Service. (2014). *2010 Population and Housing Census: Summary Report of Final Results*. Accra: Ghana Statistical Service.

Ghana Statistical Service. (2022). *2021 Population and Housing Census: General Report*. Accra: Ghana Statistical Service.

GhanaWeb. (2013). President Mahama speaks: Homosexuality is criminal. GhanaWeb, February 1. https://www.ghanaweb.com/GhanaHomePage/NewsArchive/President-Mahama-speaks-Homosexuality-is-criminal-263862

GhanaWeb. (2015). Homosexuality is not a human right—Palmer Buckle. GhanaWeb, August 1. http://www.ghananewSAGEncy.org/social/homosexuality-is-not-human-rights-palmer-buckle—92595

GhanaWeb. (2017). Legalising homosexuality "not on the agenda" but "bound to happen"—Akufo-Addo. GhanaWeb, November 26. https://www.ghanaweb.com/GhanaHomePage/NewsArchive/Legalising-homosexuality-not-on-the-agenda-but-bound-to-happen-Akufo-Addo-604072

GhanaWeb. (2018a). I will resign if Akufo-Addo legalizes homosexuality—Speaker. GhanaWeb, May 14. https://www.ghanaweb.com/GhanaHomePage/NewsArchive/I-will-resign-if-Akufo-Addo-legalizes-homosexuality-Speaker-651656

GhanaWeb. (2018b). Coalition to pray homosexual and gay out of Ghana. GhanaWeb, May 20. https://www.ghanaweb.com/GhanaHomePage/NewsArchive/Coalition-to-pray-homosexual-and-gay-out-of-Ghana-656024

Gibson-Graham, J. K. (1996). *The End of Capitalism (as We Knew It): A Feminist Critique of Political Economy*. Minneapolis: University of Minnesota Press.

Glenn, E. (1992). From servitude to service work: Historical continuities in the racial division of paid reproductive labor. *Signs* 18, 1–43.

Gosine, A. (2005). *Sex for Pleasure, Rights to Participation, and Alternatives to AIDS: Placing Sexual Minorities and/or Dissidents in Development*. Brighton: Institute of Development Studies.

Gosine, A. (2013). Murderous men. *International Feminist Journal of Politics* 15 (4), 477–93. https://doi.org/10.1080/14616742.2013.849965.

Gosine, A. (2018). Rescue and real love: Same-sex desire in international development. In C. L. Mason (ed.), *Routledge Handbook of Queer Development Studies*, 193–208. London: Taylor Francis.

Gray, S. (2011). Ghana's president will "never support" legalising homosexuality. PinkNews, March 11. http://www.pinknews.co.uk/2011/11/03/ghanas-president-will-never-support-legalising-homosexuality/

Griffin, P. (2007). Sexing the economy in a neo-liberal world order: Neo-liberal discourse and the (re)production of heteronormative heterosexuality. *British Journal of Politics and International Relations* 9 (2), 220–38.

Guerini, F. (2009). Multilingualism and language attitudes in Ghana: A preliminary survey. *Ethnorema* IV (4) 1–33.

Gyamerah, A. (2017). Unburying the ostrich's head and opening Pandora's Box: A paradigm shift to address HIV among men who have sex with men in Ghana. PhD diss., Columbia University.

Gyamerah, A. (2021). Moral panic and other unintended consequences in Ghana's paradigm shift to address HIV among men who have sex with men. In T. Sandfort (ed.), *Male Same-Sex Sexuality and HIV in Sub-Saharan Africa*, 117–37. Cham, Switzerland: Springer.

Hackett, R. (1999). The gospel of prosperity in West Africa. In R. H. Roberts (ed.), *Religion and the Transformations of Capitalism*, 199–214. London: Routledge.

Hall, S. (1978). *Policing the Crisis: Mugging, the State and Law and Order*. London: Macmillan.

Halperin, D. (1995). *Saint Foucault: Towards a Gay Hagiography*. Oxford University Press.

Han, E., and O'Mahoney, J. (2014). British colonialism and the criminalization of homosexuality. *Cambridge Review of International Affairs* 27 (2), 268–88. https://doi.org /10.1080/09557571.2013.867298

Haney, L. (2008). Competing empowerments: Gender and neoliberal punishment in the East and West. In C. Elliot (ed.) *Global empowerment of women: Responses to globalization and politicized religions*, 25–44. London: Routledge.

Haraway, D. J. (1991). *Simians, Cyborgs, and Women: The Reinvention of Nature*. New York: Routledge.

Harding, S. G. (1987). *Feminism and Methodology: Social Science Issues*. Milton Keynes: Open University Press.

Harman, S. (2015). 15 years of "war on AIDS": What impact has the global HIV/AIDS response had on the political economy of Africa? *Review of African Political Economy* 42 (145), 467–76. https://doi.org/10.1080/03056244.2015.1064370

Hartman, S. (2006). *Lose Your Mother: A Journey along the Atlantic Slave Route*. London: Macmillan.

Hendriks, T. (2021). "Making men fall": Queer power beyond anti-normativity. *Africa* 91 (3), 398–417. https://doi.10.1017/S000197202100022X

Hennessy, R. (2000). *Profit and Pleasure: Sexual Identities in Late Capitalism*. 2nd ed. London: Routledge.

Hennessy, R. (2006). Returning to reproduction queerly: Sex, labor, need. *Rethinking Marxism* 18 (3), 387–95. https://doi.org/10.1080/08935690600748074

Hickel, J. (2012). Neoliberal plague: The political economy of HIV transmission in Swaziland. *Journal of Southern African Studies*, 38:3, 513–29. https://doi.org/10.1080/03 057070.2012.699700

Hildebrandt, T., and Chua, L. (2017). Negotiating in/visibility: The political economy of lesbian activism and rights advocacy. *Development and Change* 48 (4), 639–62.

Hill-Collins, P. (1998). It's all in the family: Intersections of gender, race, and nation. *Hypatia* 13 (3), 62–82. http://www.jstor.org/stable/3810699

Hoad, N. (2007). *African Intimacies: Race, Homosexuality, and Globalization*. Minneapolis: University of Minnesota Press.

Hoskyns, C., and Rai, S. M. (2007). Recasting the global political economy: Counting women's unpaid work. *New Political Economy* 12 (3), 297–317. https://doi.org/10.10 80/13563460701485268

Hozić, A. A. (2021). Follow the bodies: Global capitalism, global war, global crisis and feminist IPE. *International Relations* 35 (1), 173-177. https://doi.org/10.1177/004711 7821992418

Human Rights Watch. (2008). *This Alien Legacy: The Origins of "Sodomy" Laws in British Colonialism*. New York: Human Rights Watch. https://www.hrw.org/sites/default/fil es/reports/lgbt1208_webwcover.pdf (accessed January 31, 2020).

Human Rights Watch. (2018). *"No Choice but to Deny Who I Am": Violence and Discrimination against LGBTI People in Ghana.* https://www.refworld.org/docid/5a69d2464.html (accessed January 31, 2020).

Human Rights Watch. (2019). Kenya: Court upholds archaic anti-homosexuality laws. *Human Rights Watch*, May 24. https://www.hrw.org/news/2019/05/24/kenya-court-upholds-archaic-anti-homosexuality-laws-0

Human Rights Watch. (2021). Ghana: LGBT activists face hardships after detention. Extreme anti-LGBT bill stokes hostility. September 20. https://www.hrw.org/news/2021/09/20/ghana-lgbt-activists-face-hardships-after-detention

Hutton, G., Wyss, K., and N'Diékhor, Y. (2003). Prioritization of prevention activities to combat the spread of HIV/AIDS in resource constrained settings: A cost-effectiveness analysis from Chad, Central Africa. *International Journal of Health Planning Management* 18, 117–36. https://doi.org/10.1002/hpm.700

Ince, O. U. (2018). *Colonial Capitalism and the Dilemmas of Liberalism.* New York: Oxford University Press.

Ingram, A. (2013). After the exception: HIV/AIDS beyond salvation and scarcity. *Antipode* 45, 436–54. https://doi.org/10.1111/j.1467-8330.2012.01008.x

International Monetary Fund (IMF). (2023). Executive board approves US$3 billion extended credit facility arrangement for Ghana. IMF Press Release No. 23/151. https://www.imf.org/en/News/Articles/2023/05/17/pr23151-ghana-imf-executive-board-approves-extended-credit-facility-arrangement-for-ghana (accessed September 24, 2023).

Isaack, W. (2017). African commission tackles sexual orientation, gender identity. Human Rights Watch, June 1. https://www.hrw.org/news/2017/06/01/african-commission-tackles-sexual-orientation-gender-identity

Issahaku, P. A. (2017). Correlates of intimate partner violence in Ghana. *Sage Open* 7 (2), 1–14. https://doi.org/10.1177/2158244017709861

Jackson, P. (2000). An explosion of Thai identities: Global queering and re-imagining queer theory. *Culture, Health and Sexuality* 2 (4), 405–24.

Jackson, P. (2009). Global queering and global queer theory: Thai [trans]genders and [homo]sexualities in world history. *Autrepart* 49 (1), 15–30.

Jacobs, S., and C. Klesse. (2013). Gender, Sexuality and Political Economy. *International Journal of Politics, Culture and Society* 27 (2), 129–52.

Jakobsen, J. (1998). Queer is? Queer does? Normativity and the problem of resistance. *GLQ: A Journal of Lesbian and Gay Studies* 4 (4), 511–36. https://doi.org/10.1215/10642684-4-4-511

Jalulah, W., and Freiku, S. (2011). Ghana: Stand up against gay rights—man of God urges Christian community. *AllAfrica*, November 4. https://allafrica.com/stories/201111070451.html

Jeffers, J. B., Dohlie, M.-B., and Lithur, N. O. (2010). *Assessment: Legal and Regulatory Framework Affecting Treatment of and Services for Most-at-Risk Populations in Ghana.* Health Policy Initiative, Task Order 1. Washington, DC: Futures Group.

Jjuuko, A., and Tabengwa, M. (2018). Expanded criminalisation of consensual same-sex relations in Africa: Contextualising recent developments. In N. Nicol et al. (eds.), *Envisioning Global LGBTI Human Rights: (Neo)colonialism, Neoliberalism, Resistance and Hope*, 63–96. London: Human Rights Consortium, Institute of Commonwealth Studies.

Johnson, C. (2011). African activists oppose cuts to Ugandan aid. *Washington Blade*, May 18. http://www.washingtonblade.com/2011/05/18/african-activists-oppose-cuts-to-ugandan-aid/

Johnston, L. G., Holman, A., Dahoma, M., Miller, L. A., Kim, E., Mussa, M., and Sabin, K. (2010). HIV risk and the overlap of injecting drug use and high-risk sexual behaviors among men who have sex with men in Zanzibar (Unguja), Tanzania. *International Journal of Drug Policy* 21 (6), 485–92. https://doi.org/10.1016/j.drugpo.2010.06.001

Jolly, S. (2000). "Queering" development: Exploring the links between same-sex sexualities, gender, and development. *Gender and Development* 8 (1), 78–88. https://doi.org/10.1080/741923414

Jolly, S. (2007). Why the development industry should get over its obsession with bad sex and start to think about pleasure. IDS Working Paper 283. Brighton: Institute of Development Studies.

Jolly, S. (2010). *Poverty and Sexuality: What Are the Connections? Overview and Literature Review*. Stockholm: Sida.

Jolly, S. (2011). Why is development work so straight? Heteronormativity in the international development industry. *Development in Practice* 21 (1), 18–28. https://doi.org/10.1080/09614524.2011.530233

Kalipeni, E., Oppong, J., and Craddock, S. (eds.). (2004). *HIV and AIDS in Africa: Beyond Epidemiology*. Oxford: Blackwell.

Kaoma, K. (2009). *Globalizing the Culture Wars: US Conservatives, African Churches, and Homophobia*. Somerville, MA: Political Research Associates.

Kapoor, I. (2015). The queer Third World. *Third World Quarterly* 36 (9), 1611–28. https://doi.org/10.1080/01436597.2015.1058148

Katz, C. (2001). Vagabond Capitalism and the Necessity of Social Reproduction. *Antipode* 33 (4), 709–28. https://doi.org/10.1111/1467-8330.00207

Kaufman, M. R., Cornish, F., Zimmerman, R. S., and Johnson, B. T. (2014). Health behavior change models for HIV prevention and AIDS care: Practical recommendations for a multi-level approach. *Journal of Acquired Immune Deficiency Syndromes* 66 (Suppl. 3), 250–58. https://doi.org/10.1097/QAI.0000000000000236

Kenworthy, N. (2017). *Mistreated: The Political Consequences of the Fight against AIDS in Lesotho*. Nashville: Vanderbilt University Press.

Kerr, R. B., and Mkandawire, P. (2012). Imaginative geographies of gender and HIV/AIDS: Moving beyond neoliberalism. *GeoJournal* 77, 459–73.

Keshavjee, S. (2014). *Blind Spot: How Neoliberalism Infiltrated Global Health*. Oakland: University of California Press.

khanna, a. (2009). Taming of the shrewd Meyeli Chhele: A political economy of development's sexual subject. *Development* 52 (1), 43–51. https://doi.org/10.1057/dev.20 08.70

khanna, a. (2011). Meyeli Chhele becomes MSM: Transformations of idioms of sexualness into epidemiological forms in India. In J. Edström (ed.), *Men and Development: Politicising Masculinities*, 47–57. London: Zed Books.

Klinken, v. A., and Obadare, E. (2018). Christianity, sexuality and citizenship in Africa: Critical intersections. *Citizenship Studies* 22 (6), 557–68. https://doi.org/10.1080/13 621025.2018.1494900

Kollman, K., and Waites, M. (2009). The global politics of lesbian, gay, bisexual and transgender human rights: An introduction. *Contemporary Politics* 15 (1), 1–17. https://doi.org/10.1080/13569770802674188

Konadu-Agyemang, K. (2000). The best of times and the worst of times: Structural adjustment programs and uneven development in Africa. The case of Ghana. *Professional Geographer* 52 (3), 469–83.

Korhonen, C., Kimani, M., Wahome, E., Otieno, F., Okall, D., Bailey, R. C., and Graham, S. M. (2018). Depressive symptoms and problematic alcohol and other substance use in 1476 gay, bisexual, and other MSM at three research sites in Kenya. *AIDS* 32 (11), 1507–15. https://doi.org/10.1097/QAD.000000000000184

Kotiswaran, P. (2011). *Dangerous Sex, Invisible Labor: Sex Work and the law in India.* Princeton, NJ: Princeton University Press.

Kropp Dakubu, M. (1997). *Korle Meets the Sea: A Sociolinguistic History of ACCRA.* Accra: Institute of African Studies University of Ghana.

Kunz, R. (2010). The crisis of social reproduction in rural Mexico: Challenging the "reprivatization of social reproduction" thesis. *Review of International Political Economy* 17 (5), 913–45. https://doi.org/10.1080/09692291003669644.

Kushwaha, S., Lalani, Y., Maina, G., Ogunbajo, A., Wilton, L., Agyarko-Poku, T., Adu-Sarkodie, Y., Boakye, F., Zhang, N., and Nelson, L. E. (2017). "But the moment they find out that you are MSM . . .": A qualitative investigation of HIV prevention experiences among men who have sex with men (MSM) in Ghana's health care system. *BMC Public Health* 17 (1), 1–18. https://doi.org/10.1186/s12889-017-4799-1

Lang, S. (2012). *NGOs, Civil Society, and the Public Sphere.* Cambridge University Press.

Laslett, B., and Brenner, J. (1989). Gender and social reproduction: Historical perspectives. *American Journal of Sociology* 105, 381–404.

LeBaron, G. (2010). The political economy of the household: Neoliberal restructuring, enclosures, and daily life. *Review of International Political Economy* 17 (5), 889–912.

Lewis, H. (2016). *The Politics of Everybody: Feminism, Queer Theory and Marxism at the Intersection.* London: Zed.

Lind, A. (2009). Governing intimacy, struggling for sexual rights: Challenging heteronormativity in the global development industry. *Development* 52 (1), 34–42. https://doi.org/10.1057/dev.2008.71

Lind, A. (2010). Introduction: Development, global governance, and sexual subjectivities. In A. Lind (ed.), *Development, Sexual Rights and Global Governance*, 1–19. London: Routledge.

Lindhardt, M. (ed.). (2015). *Pentecostalism in Africa: Presence and Impact of Pneumatic Christianity in Postcolonial Societies*. Leiden: Brill.

Liu, P. (2015). *Queer Marxism in Two Chinas*. Durham, NC: Duke University Press.

Lorde, A. (2007). *Sister Outsider: Essays and Speeches*. Berkeley, CA: Crossing Press.

Lorway, R. (2014). *Namibia's Rainbow Project: Gay Rights in an African Nation*. Bloomington: Indiana University Press.

Louw, E., and de B'Beri, B. E. (eds.). (2011). Special issue: The Afro-pessimism phenomenon. *Critical Arts* 5 (3), 335–466.

Lugones, M. (2007). Heterosexualism and the colonial/modern gender system. *Hypatia* 22 (1), 186–209.

Macharia, K. (2009). Queering african studies. Review of *African Intimacies: Race, Homosexuality, and Globalization* by Neville Hoad. *Criticism* 51 (1), 157–64.

Macharia, K. (2015). Archive and method in queer african studies. *Agenda* 29 (1), 140–46.

Macharia, K. (2016). On being area-studied: A litany of complaint. *GLQ: A Journal of Lesbian and Gay Studies* 22 (2), 183–89.

Makofane, K., Beck, J., Lubensky, M., and Ayala, G. (2014). Homophobic legislation and its impact on human security. *African Security Review* 23 (2), 186–95.

Makofane, K., Gueboguo, C., Lyons, D., and Sandfort, T. (2013). Men who have sex with men inadequately addressed in African AIDS national strategic plans. *Global Public Health* 8 (2), 129–43.

Mann, J. R., and Takyi, B. K. (2009). Autonomy, dependence or culture: Examining the impact of resources and socio-cultural processes on attitudes towards intimate partner violence in Ghana, Africa. *Journal of Family Violence* 24, 323–35.

Martínez, J., Duarte, A., and Rojas, M. J. (2021). Manufacturing moral panic: Weaponizing children to undermine gender justice and human rights. Global Philanthropy Project. https://globalphilanthropyproject.org/wp-content/uploads/2021/03/MMP-Case-Study-3-Ghana.pdf (accessed September 24, 2023).

Massad, J. (2007). *Desiring Arabs*. Chicago: University of Chicago Press.

Masvawure, T., Sandfort, T., Reddy, V., Collier, K., and Lane, T. (2015). "They think that gays have money": Gender identity and transactional sex among Black men who have sex with men in four South African townships. *Culture, Health and Sexuality* 17 (7), 891–905. https://doi.org/10.1080/13691058.2015.1007168

Matebeni, Z. (2012). *Exploring Black Lesbian Sexualities and Identity in South Africa: An Ethnography of Black Lesbian Urban Life*. Saarbrücken: Lambert Academic Publishing.

Matebeni, Z. (2014a). How not to write about queer South Africa. In Z. Matebeni (ed.), *Reclaiming Afrikan: Queer Perspectives on Sexual and Gender Identities*, 57–59. Athlone, South Africa: Modjaji Books.

Matebeni, Z. (ed.). (2014b). *Reclaiming Afrikan: Queer Perspectives on Sexual and Gender Identities*. Athlone, South Africa: Modjaj Books.

Matebeni, Z. (2017). Southern perspectives on gender relations and sexualities: A queer intervention. *Revista de antropologia* 60 (3), 26–44. https://doi.org/10.11606/2179 -0892.ra.2017.141826

Matebeni, Z., Munro, S., and Reddy, V. (2018). *Queer in Africa: LGBTQI Identities, Citizenship, and Activism.* New York: Routledge.

Matebeni, Z., and Pereira, J. (2014). Preface. In Z. Matebeni (ed.), *Reclaiming Afrikan: Queer Perspectives on Sexual and Gender Identities,* 7–10. Athlone, South Africa: Modjaji Books.

Mbembe, A. (2001). *On the Postcolony.* Berkeley: University of California Press.

McClintock, A. (1995). *Imperial Leather: Race, Gender, and Sexuality in the Colonial Context.* New York: Routledge.

McFadden, P. (2003). Sexual pleasure as feminist choice. *Feminist Africa* 2, 50–60.

McNally, D. (2017). Intersections and dialectics: Critical reconstructions in social reproduction theory. In T. Bhattacharya (ed.), *Social Reproduction Theory: Remapping Class, Recentering Oppression,* 94–112. London: Pluto Press.

Medley, A., Kennedy, C., O'Reilly, K., and Sweat, M. (2009). Effectiveness of peer education interventions for HIV prevention in developing countries: A systematic review and meta-analysis. *AIDS Education Prevention* 21 (3), 181–206. https://doi.org/10.15 21/aeap.2009.21.3.181.Effectiveness

Meiu, G. (2017). *Ethno-erotic Economies: Sexuality, Money, and Belonging in Kenya.* Chicago: University of Chicago Press.

Mendos, L. R. (ed.). (2019). *State-Sponsored Homophobia 2019: International Lesbian, Gay, Bisexual, Trans and Intersex Association.* Geneva: ILGA. https://ilga.org/downl oads/ILGA_State_Sponsored_Homophobia_2019.pdf

Meger, S. (2016). *Rape Loot Pillage: The Political Economy of Sexual Violence in Armed Conflict.* Oxford University Press.

Meyer, B. (2007). Pentecostalism and neo-liberal capitalism: Faith, prosperity and vision in African Pentecostal-Charismatic churches. *Journal for the Study of Religion* 20 (2), 5–28.

Mezzadri, A., S. Newman, and S. Stevano. (2022). Feminist global political economies of work and social reproduction. *Review of International Political Economy,* 29 (6), 1783–1803, https://doi.org/10.1080/09692290.2021.1957977

Mies, M. (1986). *Patriarchy and Accumulation on a World Scale: Women in the International Division of Labour.* London: Zed Books.

Minh-ha, T. T. (1989). *Woman, Native, Other: Writing Postcoloniality and Feminism.* Bloomington: Indiana University Press.

Mkhize, N., Bennett, J., Reddy, V., and Moletsane, R. (2012). The country we want to live in: Hate crimes and homophobia in the lives of black lesbian South Africans. Policy brief, Human Sciences Research Council. http://ecommons.hsrc.ac.za/bitst ream/handle/20.500.11910/3446/7234.pdf?sequence=1andisAllowed=y (accessed January 31, 2020).

Mohammed, W. F. (2020). Deconstructing homosexuality in Ghana. In S. N. Nyeck (ed.), *Routledge Handbook of Queer African Studies*, 167–83. New York: Routledge.

Mohanty, C. T. (2006). *Feminism without Borders: Decolonizing Theory, Practicing Solidarity*. New Delhi: Zubaan.

Molyneux, M. (2006). Mothers at the service of the new poverty agenda: The PROGRESA/Oportunidades programme in Mexico. *Social Policy and Administration* 40 (4), 425–49.

Monro, S., Matebeni, Z., and Reddy, V. (2020). LGBTQI+ people in Africa. In R. Rabaka (ed.), *Routledge Handbook of Pan-Africanism*, 171–84. London: Routledge.

Morgan, R. Z., and Wieringa, S. (2005). *Tommy Boys, Lesbian Men and Ancestral Wives: Female Same-Sex Practices in Africa*. Johannesburg: Jacana Media.

Morgensen, S. L. (2011). *Spaces Between Us: Queer Settler Colonialism and Indigenous Decolonization*. Minneapolis: University of Minnesota Press.

Mosley, P., Hudson, J., and Verschoor, A. (2004). Aid, poverty reduction and the "new conditionality." *Economic Journal* 114 (504), 217–48.

Msibi, T. (2011). The lies we have been told: On (homo) sexuality in Africa. *Africa Today* 58 (1), 55–77. https://doi.org/10.2979/africatoday.58.1.55

Msibi, T. (2016). Not crossing the line: Masculinities and homophobic violence in South Africa, *Agenda* 23 (80), 50–54.

Mudimbe, V. Y. (1988). *The Invention of Africa: Gnosis, Philosophy and the Order of knowledge*. Bloomington: Indiana University Press.

Müller, A., and Daskilewicz, K. (2018). Mental health among lesbian, gay, bisexual, transgender and intersex people in East and southern Africa. *European Journal of Public Health* 28 (4). https://doi.org/10.1093/eurpub/cky213.794

Muñoz, J. E. (2009). *Cruising Utopia: The Then and There of Queer Futurity*. New York: NYU Press.

Murgo, M. A. J., Huynh, K. D., Lee, D. L., and Chrisler, J. C. (2017). Anti-effeminacy moderates the relationship between masculinity and internalized heterosexism among gay men. *Journal of LGBTI Issues in Counseling* 11 (2), 106–18. https://doi.org /10.1080/15538605.2017.1310008

Murray, S., and Roscoe, W. (eds.). (1998). *Boy-Wives and Female Husbands: Studies in African Homosexualities*. New York: Palgrave Macmillan.

MyJoyOnline. (2011). BNI investigates homosexuality in Western, Central Regions. MyJoyOnline, June 1. https://www.myjoyonline.com/bni-investigates-homosexuali ty-in-western-central-regions/

MyJoyOnline. (2013). Angry Tamale youth, chief threaten to lynch homosexuals. MyJoyOnline, March 18. http://edition.myjoyonline.com/pages/news/201303/102928.php

Naidu, S., and Ossome, L. (2016). Social reproduction and the agrarian question of women's labour in India. *Agrarian South: Journal of Political Economy* 5 (1), 50–76. https://doi.org/10.1177/2277976016658737.

Nattrass, N. (2014). *The Moral Economy of AIDS in South Africa*. Cambridge University Press.

Ndashe, S. (2013). The single story of "African homophobia" Is dangerous for LGBTI activism. In S. Ekine and H. Abbas (eds.), Queer African Reader, 155–64. Nairobi: Pambazuka Press.

Ndjio, B. (2012). Post-colonial histories of sexuality: The political invention of a libidinal African straight. Africa 82 (4), 609–31. https://doi.org/10.1017/S0001972012000526

Ndjio, B. (2013). Sexuality and nationalist ideologies in post-colonial Cameroon. In S. Wieringa and H. Sívori (eds.), The Sexual History of the Global South: Sexual Politics in Africa, Asia and Latin America, 120–43. London: Zed Books.

Ndoye, A. S. and Onekekou, E. (2019). The situation of the LGBTI community in West Africa. In R. Mendos (ed.), State-Sponsored Homophobia 2019: International Lesbian, Gay, Bisexual, Trans and Intersex Association, 89–91. Geneva: ILGA.

Nettey, J. (2018). Police save suspected lesbians from lynching. Herald Ghana, February 14. http://theheraldghana.com/police-save-suspected-lesbians-from-lynching/

Nguyen, V. K. (2005). Uses and pleasures: Sexual modernity, HIV/AIDS, and confessional technologies in a West African metropolis. In V. Adams and S. L. Pigg (eds.), Sex in Development: Science, Sexuality, and Morality in Global Perspective, 245–68. Durham, NC: Duke University Press.

Nguyen, V. K. (2010). The Republic of Therapy: Triage and Sovereignty in West Africa's Time of AIDS. Durham, NC: Duke University Press.

Nketiah, R. (2019). "God has a new Africa": Undercover in a US-led anti-LGBT "hate movement." Open Democracy, December 11. https://www.opendemocracy.net/en/5050/god-has-a-new-africa-undercover-in-a-us-led-anti-lgbt-hate-movement/

Nkrumah, K. (1965). Neocolonialism: The Last Stage of Imperialism. London: Thomas Nelson and Sons Ltd.

Nyanzi, S. (2013). Dismantling reified African culture through localised homosexualities in Uganda. Culture, Health and Sexuality 15 (8), 952–67.

Nyanzi, S. (2014). Queering queer Africa. In Z. Matebeni (ed.), Reclaiming Afrikan: Queer Perspectives on Sexual and Gender Identities, 65–69. Athlone, South African: Modjaji Books.

Nyanzi, S. (2015). Knowledge is requisite power: Making a case for queer African scholarship. In T. Sandfort, F. Simenel, K. Mwachiro, and V. Reddy (eds.), Boldly Queer: African Perspectives on Same-Sex Sexuality and Gender Diversity, 125–35. The Hague: HIVOS.

Nyanzi, S., and Karamagi, A. (2015). The social-political dynamics of the anti-homosexuality legislation in Uganda. Agenda 950, 1–15.

Nyato, D., Kuringe, E., Drake, M., Casalini, C., Nnko, S., Shao, A., and Changalucha, J. (2018). Participants' accrual and delivery of HIV prevention interventions among men who have sex with men in sub-Saharan Africa: A systematic review. BMC Public Health 18 (1). https://doi.org/10.1186/s12889-018-5303-2

Nyeck, S. N. (2013). Mobilizing against the invisible: Erotic nationalism, mass media, and the "paranoid style" in Cameroon. In S. N. Nyeck and M. Epprecht (eds.), Sexual Diversity in Africa: Politics, Theory, and Citizenship, 151–69. Montreal: McGill-Queen's University Press.

Nyeck, S. N. (ed.). (2020). *Routledge Handbook of Queer African Studies*. London: Routledge.

Nyeck, S. N. (2021). *African(a) Queer Presence: Ethics and Politics of Negotiation*. New York: Palgrave Macmillan.

Nyeck, S. N., and Epprecht, M. (eds.). (2013). *Sexual Diversity in Africa: Politics, Theory, and Citizenship*. Montreal: McGill-Queen's University Press.

Obadare-Onyango, M. A., Adu-Sarkodie, Y., Agyarko-Poku, T., Asafo, M. K., Sylvester, J., Wondergem, P., and Beard, J. (2015). "It's all about making a life": Poverty, HIV, violence, and other vulnerabilities faced by young female sex workers in Kumasi, Ghana. *Journal of Acquired Immune Deficiency Syndromes* 68, S131–S137. https://doi .org/10.1097/QAI.0000000000000455

Obeng-Odoom, F. (2012). Neoliberalism and the urban economy in Ghana: Urban employment, inequality, and poverty. *Growth and Change* 43, 85–109. https://doi .org/10.1111/j.1468-2257.2011.00578.x

Okanlawon, K. (2015). Resisting the hypocritical Western narrative of and celebrating the resistance against homophobia. In T. Sandfort et al. (eds.), *Boldly Queer: African Perspectives on Same-Sex Sexuality and Gender Diversity*, 103–16. The Hague: HIVOS.

Okertchiri, J. A. (2012). Ghana—Clash over gay rights. actup.org, March 31. http://actup .org/news/ghana-clash-over-gay-rights/

Okoye, V. (2010). Report from the field—Trotro: An essential mode of transport in Accra. *State of the Planet* blog, Earth Institute, Columbia University. https://blogs.ei .columbia.edu/2010/09/29/report-from-the-field-the-tro-tro-an-essential-mode-of -transport-in-accra-ghana/ (accessed January 31, 2020).

O'Laughlin, B. (2015). Trapped in the prison of the proximate: structural HIV/AIDS prevention in southern Africa. *Review of African Political Economy*, 42 (145), 342–61. https://doi.org/10.1080/03056244.2015.1064368

O'Laughlin, B. (2022). No separate spheres: The contingent reproduction of living labor in southern Africa. *Review of International Political Economy* 29 (6), 1827–46. https://doi.org/10.1080/09692290.2021.1950025

Oluoch, A., and Tabengwa, M. (2017). LGBTI visibility: A double-edged sword. In A. Carroll and L. R. Mendos, *State-Sponsored Homophobia 2016: A World Survey of Sexual Orientation Laws. Criminalisation, Protection and Recognition*, 150–54. Geneva: ILGA.

O'Mara, K. (2007). Homophobia and building queer community in urban Ghana. *Phoebe: Journal of Gender and Cultural Critiques* 19 (1), 35–46.

O'Mara, K. (2013). LGBTI community and citizenship practices in urban Ghana. In S. N. Nyeck and M. Epprecht (eds.), *Sexual Diversity in Africa: Politics, Theory, and Citizenship*, 188–207. Montreal: McGill-Queen's University Press.

Opare, J. A. (2003). *Kayayei*: The women head porters of southern Ghana. *Journal of Social Development in Africa* 18 (2), 33–48.

Organization for Economic Cooperation and Development. (2015). *Development Aid at a Glance, Statistics by Region, 2. Africa.* http://www.oecd.org/dac/stats/documentup load/2Africa—DevelopmentAidataGlance2016.pdf (accessed May 17, 2023).

Osei, A. (2018). Parliament has spoken, the gay question is settled. GhanaWeb, June 20. https://www.ghanaweb.com/GhanaHomePage/features/Parliament-has-spoken -the-gay-question-is-settled-661629

Ossome, L. (2021). The care economy and the state in Africa's Covid-19 responses. *Canadian Journal of Development Studies / Revue canadienne d'études du développement* 42 (1–2), 68–78. https://doi.org/10.1080/02255189.2020.1831448

Oswin, N. (2007). Producing homonormativity in neoliberal South Africa: Recognition, redistribution, and the equality project. *Signs* 32 (3), 649–69. https://doi.org/10.10 86/510337

Otu, K. (2022). *Amphibious Subjects: Sasso and the Contested Politics of Queer Self-Making in Neoliberal Ghana.* Berkeley: University of California Press.

Oyěwùmí, O. (1997). *The Invention of Women: Making an African Sense of Western Gender Discourses.* Minneapolis: University of Minnesota Press.

Pambazuka News. (2011). Statement on British "aid cut" threats to African countries that violate LBGTI rights. Pambazuka News, October 27. https://www.pambazuka.org /activism/statement-british-aid-cut-threats-african-countries-violate-lbgti-rights

Park, A. (2016). A development agenda for sexual and gender minorities. Williams Institute, UCLA School of Law. https://williamsinstitute.law.ucla.edu/wp-content/uploa ds/Development-Agenda-SGM-Jul-2016.pdf (accessed May 4, 2023),

Parpart, J. L., Rai, S., and Staudt, K. (2002). *Rethinking Empowerment: Gender and Development in a Global-Local World.* London: Routledge.

Parreñas, R. S. (2000). Migrant Filipina Domestic Workers and the International Division of Reproductive Labor. *Gender and Society* 14 (4), 560–80. https://doi.org/10.11 77/089124300014004005

Paternotte, D. (2020). Backlash: A misleading narrative. LSE Engenderings, March 30. https://blogs.lse.ac.uk/gender/2020/03/30/backlash-a-misleading-narrative/

Petchesky, R. P. (2000). Reproductive and sexual rights: Charting the course of transnational women's NGOs. Geneva 2000 Occasional Paper No. 8. Geneva: United Nations Research Institute for Social Development.

Peterson, V. S. (2003). *A Critical Rewriting of Global Political Economy: Integrating Reproductive, Productive and Virtual Economies.* London: Routledge.

Peterson, V. S. (2005). How (the meaning of) gender matters in political economy. *New Political Economy* 10 (4), 499-521. https://doi.org/10.1080/13563460500344468

Peterson, V. S. (2014a). Sex matters: A queer history of hierarchies. *International Feminist Journal of Politics* 16 (3), 389–409. https://doi.org/10.1080/14616742.2014.91 3384

Peterson, V. S. (2014b). Family matters: How queering the intimate queers the international. *International Studies Review* 16 (4), 604–8. https://doi.org/10.1111/misr .12185

Pew Research Center. (2013). *The Global Divide on Homosexuality: Greater Acceptance in More Secular and Affluent Countries*. Washington, DC: Pew Research Center.

Pew Research Center. (2014). *Morality Interactive Topline Results*. Washington, DC: Pew Research Center.

Pierre, J. (2012). *The Predicament of Blackness: Postcolonial Ghana and the Politics of Race*. Chicago: University of Chicago Press.

Pilkey, B. (2014). Queering heteronormativity at home: Older gay Londoners and the negotiation of domestic materiality *Gender, Place and Culture* 21 (9), 1142–57.

Pinfold, C. (2013). Ghana: Anti-gay critics say new children's minister will "promote homosexuality." *PinkNews*, April 2. http://www.pinknews.co.uk/2013/02/04/ghana -anti-gay-critics-say-new-childrens-minister-will-promote-homosexuality/

Pinkerton, S., Holtgrave, D., DiFranceisco, W., Stevenson, L., and Kelly, J. (1998). Cost-effectiveness of a community-level HIV risk reduction intervention. *American Journal of Public Health* 88 (8), 1239–42.

Population Council. (2000). *Peer Education and HIV/AIDS: Past Experience, Future Directions*. Washington, DC: Population Council.

Puar, J. K. (2002). Circuits of queer mobility: Tourism, travel, and globalization. *GLQ: A Journal of Lesbian and Gay Studies* 8 (1), 101–37.

Puar, J. K (2007). *Terrorist Assemblages: Homonationalism in Queer Times*, Durham, NC: Duke University Press.

Puar, J. K. (2013). Rethinking homonationalism. *International Journal of Middle East Studies* 45 (2), 336–39. https://doi.org/10.1017/S002074381300007X

Puri, J. K. (2016). *Sexual States: Governance and the Struggle over the Antisodomy Law in India*. Durham, NC: Duke University Press.

Rai, S. (2002). *Gender and the Political Economy of Development: From Nationalism to Globalization*. London: Polity Press.

Rai, S., and Waylen, G. (eds.) (2008). *Global Governance: Feminist Perspectives*. Basingstoke: Palgrave Macmillan.

Ransby, B. (2017). Fortieth anniversary of the Combahee River Collective Statement. In K.-Y. Taylor (ed.), *How We Get Free: Black Feminism and the Combahee River Collective*, 177–84. New York: Haymarket Books.

Rao, R. (2014). The locations of homophobia. *London Review of International Law* 2 (2), 169–99.

Rao, R. (2015). Global homocapitalism. *Radical Philosophy* 194, 38–49.

Rao, R. (2020). *Out of Time: The Queer Politics of Postcoloniality*. Oxford University Press.

Reddy, V., Monro, S., and Matebeni, Z. (2018). Introduction. In Z. Matebeni, S. Monro, and V. Reddy (eds.), *Queer in Africa LGBTQI Identities, Citizenship, and Activism*, 1–16. London: Routledge.

Reid, G., and Dirsuweit, T. (2002). Understanding systemic violence: Homophobic attacks in Johannesburg. *Urban Forum* 13, 99–126.

Reuters. (2021). Ghana president calls for tolerance as parliament considers anti-LGBT+ law. Reuters, October 22. https://www.reuters.com/world/africa/ghana-president-calls-tolerance-parliament-considers-anti-lgbt-law-2021-10-21/

Rightify Ghana (2021). In 2019, when World Congress of Families held a regional conference in Ghana, they prepared grounds for the anti-LGBTQ bill. World Congress of Families enabled and promoted legislation to further criminalize LGBTQ people, including in Nigeria and Uganda. 12.37 p.m., July 1. Tweet. https://twitter.com/RightifyGhana/status/1410563294834929671

Rioux, S. (2015). Embodied Contradictions: Capitalism, Social Reproduction and Body Formation. *Women's Studies International Forum* 48 (1), 194–202. https://doi.org/10.1016/j.wsif.2014.03.008.

Roberts, A. (2015). Gender, financial deepening and the production of embodied finance: Towards a critical feminist analysis. *Global Society* 29 (1), 107–27. https://doi.org/10.1080/13600826.2014.975189

Roberts, A., and Soederberg, S. (2012). Gender equality as *smart economics*? A critique of the 2012 *World Development Report*. *Third World Quarterly* 33 (5), 949–68. https://doi.org/10.1080/01436597.2012.677310

Roberts, M. (1995). Emergence of gay identity and gay social movements in developing Countries: The AIDS crisis as catalyst. *Alternatives: Global, Local, Political* 20 (2), 243–64.

Robertson, J. (2009). CEPEHRG and Maritime, Ghana: Engaging new partners and new technologies to prevent HIV among men who have sex with men. AIDSTAR One, Arlington, VA. http://www.aidstarUone.com/sites/default/files/AIDSTARUOne_Case_Study_MSM_Ghana_lowres_updated_0.pdf (accessed January 31, 2020).

Rodney, W. (1972). *How Europe Underdeveloped Africa*. London: Bogle-L'Ouverture Publications.

Rodriguez, S. M. (2017). Homophobic nationalism: the development of sodomy legislation in Uganda. *Comparative Sociology* 16 (3), 393–421. https://doi.org/10.1163/15691330-12341430

Rodriguez, S. M. (2019). *The Economies of Queer Inclusion: Transnational Organizing for LGBTI Rights in Uganda*. Lanham, MD: Lexington Books.

Roy, A. (2014). The NGO-ization of resistance. Massalijn, September 4. http://massalijn.nl/new/the-ngo-ization-of-resistance

Ruckert, A. (2010). The forgotten dimension of social reproduction: The World Bank and the poverty reduction strategy paradigm. *Review of International Political Economy* 17 (5), 816–39. https://doi.org/10.1080/09692291003712113

Sánchez, F. J., Blas-Lopez, F. J., Martínez-Patiño, M. J., and Vilain, E. (2016). Masculine consciousness and anti-effeminacy among Latino and White gay men. *Psychology of Men and Masculinity* 17 (1), 54–63. https://doi.org/10.1037/a0039465

Sánchez, F. J., and Vilain, E. (2012). "Straight-acting gays": The relationship between masculine consciousness, anti-effeminacy, and negative gay identity. *Archives of Sexual Behavior* 41, 111–19. https://doi.org/10.1007/s10508-012-9912-z

Sandfort, T., Simenel, F., Mwachiro, K., and Reddy, V. (eds.). (2015). *Boldly Queer: African Perspectives on Same-Sex Sexuality and Gender Diversity*. The Hague, NL: HIVOS.

Scheibe, A., Kanyemba, B., Syvertsen, J., Adebajo, S., and Baral, S. (2014). Money, power and HIV: Economic influences and HIV among men who have sex with men in sub-Saharan Africa. *African Journal of Reproductive Health* 18 (3), 84–92.

Schulman, S. (2011). Israel and "pinkwashing." *New York Times*, November 22. https://www.nytimes.com/2011/11/23/opinion/pinkwashing-and-israels-use-of-gays-as-a-messaging-tool.html

Sears, A. (2017). Body politics: The social reproduction of sexualities. In T. Bhattacharya (ed.), *Social Reproduction Theory: Remapping Class, Recentering Oppression*, 171–91. London: Pluto Press.

Shaban, A. (2018). Ghana president says he will never oversee same-sex legalization. AfricaNews, April 30. https://www.africanews.com/2018/04/30/ghana-president-says-he-will-never-oversee-same-sex-legalization/

Sharma, A. (2008). *Logics of Empowerment: Development, Gender, and Governance in Neoliberal India*. Minneapolis: University of Minnesota Press.

Shepard, B. H. (1997). *White Nights and Ascending Shadows: An Oral History of the San Francisco AIDS Epidemic*. Washington, DC: Cassell.

Shipley, J. (2009). Comedians, pastory, and the miraculous agency of charisma in Ghana. *Cultural Anthropology* 24 (3), 523–52.

Smith, A. D., Tapsoba, P., Peshu, N., Sanders, E. J., and Jaffe, H. W. (2009). Men who have sex with men and HIV/AIDS in sub-Saharan Africa. *The Lancet* 374 (9687), 416–22. https://doi.org/10.1016/S0140-6736(09)61118-1

Smith, B. (2019). Why I left the mainstream queer rights movement. *New York Times*, June 19. https://www.nytimes.com/2019/06/19/us/barbara-smith-black-queer-rights.html

Smith, L. T. (1999). *Decolonizing Methodologies: Research and Indigenous Peoples*. New York: Zed Books.

Smith, N. (2012). Body issues: The political economy of male sex work. *Sexualities* 15 (5–6), 586–603. https://doi.org/10.1177/1363460712445983

Smith, N. (2016). Toward a queer political economy of crisis. In J. True and A. Hozić (eds.), *Scandalous Economics: The Politics of Gender and Financial Crises*, 231–47. New York: Oxford University Press.

Smith, N. (2018). Queer theory and feminist political economy. In J. Elias and A. Roberts (eds.), *Handbook on the International Political Economy of Gender*, 102–12. London: Edward Elgar.

Smith, N. (2020). *Capitalism's Sexuality History*. Oxford University Press.

Snorton, C. R. (2017). *Black on Both Sides: A Racial History of Trans Identity*. Minneapolis: University of Minnesota Press.

Soothill, J. (2007). *Gender, Social Change and Spiritual Power: Charismatic Christianity in Ghana*. Boston: Brill.

Spillers, H. J. (1987). Mama's Baby, Papa's Maybe: An American Grammar Book. *Diacritics*, 17 (2), 65–81. https://doi.org/10.2307/464747

Spivak, G. (1988). Can the subaltern speak? In C. Nelson and L. Grossberg (eds.), *Marxism and the Interpretation of Culture*, 271–316. Urbana: University of Illinois Press.

Spronk, R., and Hendriks, T. (2020). *Readings in Sexualities from Africa*. Bloomington: Indiana University Press.

Spronk, R., and Nyeck, S. N. (2021). Frontiers and pioneers in (the study of) queer experiences in Africa: Introduction. *Africa* 91 (3), 388–97. https://doi.org/10.1017/S000 1972021000231

Ssebaggala, R. (2011). Straight talk on the gay question in Uganda. *Transition* 57 (106), 44–57. https://doi.org/10.2979/transition.106b.44

Steans, J. (2003). Engaging from the Margins: Feminist encounters with the "mainstream" of international relations. *British Journal of Politics and International Relations* 5 (3), 428–54.

Steans, J., and Tepe, D. (2008). Gender in the theory and practice of international political economy: The promise and limitations of neo-Gramscian approaches. In A. J. Ayers (ed.), *Gramsci, Political Economy, and International Relations Theory: Modern Princes and Naked Emperors*, 133–52. New York: Palgrave Macmillan.

Stoler, A. L. (2002). *Carnal Knowledge and Imperial Power: Race and the Intimate in Colonial Rule*. Oakland: University of California Press.

Strange, V., Forrest, S., and Oakley, A. (2002). Peer-led sex education-characteristics of peer educators and their perceptions of the impact on them of participation in a peer education programme. *Health Education Research* 17 (3), 327–37.

Swarr, A. L. (2012). *Sex in Transition: Remaking Gender and Race in South Africa*. Albany: SUNY Press.

Takyi, B. K., and Mann, J. R. (2006). Intimate partner violence in Ghana: The perspectives of men regarding wife beating. *International Journal of Sociology of the Family* 32, 61–78.

Tamale, S. (2003). Out of the closet: Unveiling sexuality discourses in Uganda. *Feminist Africa* 2 (2), 1–6.

Tamale, S. (ed.). (2011). *African Sexualities: A Reader*. Cape Town: Pambazuka Press.

Tamale, S. (2013). Confronting the politics of nonconforming sexualities in Africa. *African Studies Review* 56 (2), 31–45.

Tamale, S. (2020). *Decolonization and Afro-Feminism*. Montreal: Daraja Press.

Taylor Williamson, R., Wondergem, P, and Amenyah, R. (2014). Using a reporting system to protect the human rights of people living with HIV and key populations: A conceptual framework. *Health and Human Rights Journal* 1 (16), 148–56.

Taywaditep, K. J. (2002). Marginalization among the marginalized. *Journal of Homosexuality* 42 (1), 1–28. https://doi.org/10.1300/J082v42n01

Tellis, A., and Bala, S. (eds.). (2015). *The Global Trajectories of Queerness: Re-thinking Same-Sex Politics in the Global South*. Leiden: Brill.

Tettey, W. J. (2016). Homosexuality, moral panic, and politicized homophobia in Ghana: Interrogating discourses of moral entrepreneurship in Ghanaian media. *Communication, Culture and Critique* 9 (1), 86–106. https://doi.org/10.1111/cccr.12132

Theron, L., McAllister, J., and Armisen, M. (2016). Where do we go from here? A call for critical reflection on queer/LGBTIA+ activism in Africa. *Pambazuka News*, May 12. https://www.pambazuka.org/gender-minorities/where-do-we-go-here

Thomann, M. (2014). The price of inclusion: Sexual subjectivity, violence, and the non-profit industrial complex in Abidjan, Côte d'Ivoire. PhD diss., American University.

Thoreson, R. R. (2009). Queering human rights: The Yogyakarta principles and the norm that dare not speak its name. *Journal of Human Rights* 8 (4), 323–39. https://doi.org/10.1080/14754830903324746

Thoreson, R. R. (2014). Troubling the waters of a "wave of homophobia": Political economies of anti-queer animus in sub-Saharan Africa. *Sexualities* 17 (1–2), 23–42. https://doi.org/10.1177/1363460713511098

Tilley, L., and Shilliam, R. (2018). Raced markets: An introduction. *New Political Economy* 23 (5), 534–43. https://doi.org/10.1080/13563467.2017.1417366

Tran, V. (2011). Sexuality and gender law clinic secures asylum for gay Mauritanian refugee. *Gender and Sexuality* blog, Columbia Law School, October 26. http://blogs.law.columbia.edu/genderandsexualitylawblog/2011/10/26/sexuality-and-gender-law-clinic-secures-asylum-for-gay-mauritanian-refugee/

True, J. (2012). *The Political Economy of Violence against Women*. Oxford University Press.

Tsikata, D. (2009). Women's organizing in Ghana since the 1990s: From individual organizations to three coalitions. *Development* 52 (2), 185–92.

Turner, G., and Shepherd, J. (1999). A method in search of a theory: Peer education and health promotion. *Health Education Research* 14 (2), 235–47. https://doi.org/10.1093/her/14.2.235

United Nations Program on HIV/AIDS (UNAIDS). (1999). *Peer Education and HIV/AIDS*. Washington, DC: UNAIDS.

United Nations Program on HIV/AIDS (UNAIDS). (2015). *Terminology Guidelines*. Washington, DC: UNAIDS.

United Nations Program on HIV/AIDS (UNAIDS). (2018). *UNAIDS Data 2018*. Washington, DC: UNAIDS.

US Agency for International Development (USAID). (2013). The USAID vision for action: Promoting and supporting the inclusion of lesbian, gay, bisexual, and transgender individuals. December. http://www.usaid.gov/sites/default/files/Draft_USAID_LGBT_Vision_for_Public_Comment.pdf (accessed May 17, 2023).

US Agency for International Development (USAID). (2019). Country profile: Ghana. https://idea.usaid.gov/cd/ghana?comparisonGroup=region (accessed May 17, 2023).

Valenza, A. (2011). Ghana: The Coalition Against Homophobia in Ghana (CAHG) educate people about respect for LGBTI rights. ILGA, August 8. http://ilga.org/ghana-thecoalition-against-homophobia-in-ghana-cahg-educate-people-about-respect-for-lgbti-rights/

Valocchi, S. (2017). Capitalisms and gay identities: Towards a capitalist theory of social movements. *Social Problems* 64 (2), 315–31. https://www.jstor.org/stable/26370910

Vibe Ghana. (2011). Ghana's president slams David Cameron: You can't threaten us with gay aid. Vibe Ghana, November 2. http://vibeghana.com/2011/11/02/ghanas-presid ent-slams-david-cameron-you-cant-threaten-us-with-gay-aid/

Vibe Ghana. (2012). Woman marries woman in Ghana. Vibe Ghana, March 19. http://vi beghana.com/2012/03/19/woman-marries-woman-in-ghana

Vider, S. (2014). "Oh hell, May, why don't you people have a cookbook?": Camp humor and gay domesticity. *American Quarterly* 65 (4), 877–904.

Vogel, L. ([1983] 2013). *Marxism and the Oppression of Women: Toward a Unitary Theory*. New Brunswick, NJ: Rutgers University Press.

Vrede, K. (2020). Fighting the power: Queer social movements and their impact on African laws and culture. *Cornell International Law Journal* 53 (3), 467–96.

Wainaina, B. ([2005] 2019). How to write about Africa. *Granta* 92, May 2. https://granta .com/how-to-write-about-africa/

Walia, H. (2022). *Border and Rule: Global Migration, Capitalism, and the Rise of Racist Nationalism*. Chicago: Haymarket Books.

Wallace, A., Maulbeck, B., and Kan, L. (2018). *2015/2016 Resources Report: Government and Philanthropic Support for Lesbian, Gay, Bisexual, Transgender, and Intersex Communities*. N.p.: Funders for LGBTQ Issues.

Ward, K. (2013). Religious institutions and actors and religious attitudes to homosexual rights: South Africa and Uganda. In C. Lennox and M. Waites (eds.), *Human Rights, Sexual Orientation and Gender Identity in the Commonwealth: Struggles for Decriminalisation and Change*, 409–10. London: Institute of Commonwealth Studies.

Waylen, G. (1997). Gender, feminism and political economy. *New Political Economy* 2 (2), 205–20.

Waylen, G. (2006). You still don't understand: Why troubled engagements continue between feminists and (critical) IPE. *Review of International Studies* 32 (1), 145–64.

Weber, C. 2016. *Queer International Relations: Sovereignty, Sexuality and the Will to Knowledge*. New York: Oxford University Press.

Weeks, J. (2000). *Making Sexual History*. London: Polity Press.

Weeks, J. (2003). *Sexuality: Key Ideas*. London: Routledge.

Wekker, G. (2006). *The Politics of Passion: Women's Sexual Culture in the Afro-Surinamese Diaspora*. New York: Columbia University Press.

Wiegman, R., and Wilson, E. (2015). Introduction: Antinormativity's queer conventions. *differences* 26 (1), 1–25. https://doi.org/10.1215/10407391-2880582

Wilson, K. (2015). Towards a radical re-appropriation: gender, development and neoliberal feminism. *Development and Change* 46, 803–32. https://doi.org/10.1111/de ch.12176

World Health Organization. (2012). *Prevention and Treatment of HIV and Other Sexually Transmitted Infections for Sex Workers in Low-and Middle-Income Countries*. Geneva: WHO. http://www.who.int/hiv/pub/guidelines/sex_worker/en/index.html (accessed January 30, 2020).

World Health Organization. (2016). FAQ on health and sexual diversity: An introduction to key concepts. Geneva: WHO. https://iris.who.int/bitstream/handle/10665/255340/WHO-FWC-GER-16.2-eng.pdf?sequence=1

World Health Organization. (2017). *Sexual Health and Its Linkages to Reproductive Health: An Operational Approach*. Geneva: WHO.

Wright, T. (2000). Gay organizations, NGOS, and the globalization of sexual identity: The case of Bolivia. *Journal of Latin American Anthropology* 5, 89–111. https://doi-org.manchester.idm.oclc.org/10.1525/jlca.2000.5.2.89

Yang, D. (2019). Global trends on the decriminalisation of consensual same-sex sexual acts (1969–2019). In R. Mendos (ed.), *State-Sponsored Homophobia 2019: International Lesbian, Gay, Bisexual, Trans and Intersex Association*, 175–96. Geneva: ILGA.

Ye, S. (2021). "Paris" and "scar": Queer social reproduction, homonormative division of labour and HIV/AIDS economy in postsocialist China. *Gender, Place and Culture* 28 (12), 1778–98. https://doi.org/10.1080/0966369X.2021.1873742

Yogyakarta Principles. (2007). Principles on the application of international human rights law in relation to sexual orientation and gender identity. https://yogyakartaprinciples.org/ (accessed January 31, 2020).

Youngs, G. (ed.) (2000). *Political Economy, Power and the Body: Global Perspectives*. Basingstoke: Palgrave Macmillan.

Yussif, A. S., Amoafo, R. A., and Adomako, K. (2016). Lesbian, gay, bisexual, and transgender intersex and queer (LGBTIQ) people in Ghana: Joint stakeholder report by the working group of CSOs. Accra: Solace Foundation (accessed November 28, 2023).